OXFORD MEDICAL PUBLICATIONS

Healthy Skin

THE FACTS

ALSO PUBLISHED BY OXFORD
UNIVERSITY PRESS

Ageing: the facts (second edition)
Nicholas Coni, William Davison,
and Stephen Webster

Alcoholism: the facts
Donald W. Goodwin

Allergy: the facts
Robert J. Davies and Susan Ollier

**Arthritis and rheumatism:
the facts**
J. T. Scott

Asthma: the facts (second edition)
Donald J. Lane and Anthony Storr

Back pain: the facts
(second edition)
Malcolm Jayson

Blood disorders: the facts
Sheila T. Callender

Breast cancer: the facts
(second edition) Michael Baum

Cancer: the facts
Sir Ronald Bodley Scott

Childhood diabetes: the facts
J. O. Craig

Contraception: the facts
(second edition)
Peter Bromwich and Tony Parsons

**Coronary heart disease:
the facts** (second edition)
Desmond Julian and Claire Marley

Cystic fibrosis: the facts
(second edition)
Ann Harris and Maurice Super

Deafness: the facts
Andrew P. Freeland

Down syndrome: the facts
Mark Selikowitz

Eating disorders: the facts
(third edition)
Suzanne Abraham and Derek
Llewellyn-Jones

Epilepsy: the facts
Anthony Hopkins

Head injury: the facts
Dorothy Gronwall, Philip
Wrightson, and Peter Waddell

Healthy skin: the facts
Rona M. MacKie

Hypothermia: the facts
K. J. Collins

Kidney disease: the facts
(second edition) Stewart Cameron

**Liver disease and gallstones:
the facts**
A. G. Johnson and D. Triger

Lung cancer: the facts
(second edition) Chris Williams

Migraine: the facts
F. Clifford Rose and M. Gawel

Miscarriage: the facts
G. C. L. Lachelin

Multiple sclerosis: the facts
(second edition) Bryan Matthews

**Obsessive–compulsive disorder:
the facts**
Padmal de Silva and S. Rachman

Parkinson's disease: the facts
(second edition)
Gerald Stern and Andrew Lees

Pre-eclampsia: the facts
Chris Redman and Isabel Walker

Rabies: the facts
(second edition) Colin Kaplan,
G. S. Turner, and D. A. Warrell

**Sexually transmitted diseases:
the facts**
David Barlow

Stroke: the facts
F. Clifford Rose and R. Capildeo

Thyroid disease: the facts
(second edition) R. I. S. Bayliss and
W. M. G. Tunbridge

Healthy Skin

THE FACTS

RONA M. MacKIE

Professor of Dermatology
University of Glasgow

Consultant Dermatologist
Greater Glasgow Health Board
Western Infirmary Glasgow and
Royal Hospital for Sick Children
Glasgow

OXFORD   NEW YORK   TOKYO
OXFORD UNIVERSITY PRESS
1992

Oxford University Press, Walton Street, Oxford OX2 6DP
Oxford New York Toronto
Delhi Bombay Calcutta Madras Karachi
Petaling Jaya Singapore Hong Kong Tokyo
Nairobi Dar es Salaam Cape Town
Melbourne Auckland
and associated companies in
Berlin Ibadan

Oxford is a trade mark of Oxford University Press

Published in the United States
by Oxford University Press, New York

A catalogue record for this book is available from the British Library

Library of Congress Cataloging in Publication Data
MacKie, Rona M.
Healthy skin : the facts : good skin care throughout life / Rona
M. MacKie
Includes index.
1. Skin—Care and hygiene.   I. Title.   II. Series.   III. Series:
Facts/OPB
[DNLM: 1. Skin—physiology—popular works.   2. Skin Aging—popular
works.   3. Skin Diseases—popular works.   WR 140 M158]
RL87.M24   1992
616.5—dc20   91-39238

ISBN 0-19-262244-7 (pbk.)
ISBN 0-19-262246-3 (hb.)

Typeset by Cambridge Composing (UK) Ltd
Printed and bound in Hong Kong

Preface

Most people never think about their skin. We can all see that it is there, but it may not seem particularly exciting or interesting—until something goes wrong. However, skin problems have a much lower profile than, for example, heart disease, probably because the skin is visible, and is not a hidden, mysterious organ like the heart or the liver, which has to be visualized with special equipment.

Healthy skin is essential to our well-being—both physical and psychological. Anyone who has a chronic skin disease—eczema or psoriasis, for example—will know that coping in normal everyday life with a visible and uncomfortable skin problem is difficult and depressing.

Few people realise the vast numbers of people who suffer from skin diseases, or that the most common form of cancer worldwide is skin cancer. Long before skin cancers develop, older people who are at increased risk of developing such problems have the inconvenience of a dry, irritable, uncomfortable skin, particularly if they have not looked after their skin adequately in their younger days. Many skin problems, including skin cancer, can be prevented by a sensible skin care routine, developed in early adult life.

Quite apart from the issue of actual skin disease, it is through the skin that we communicate with the outside world. Caring for the skin is not unnecessary vanity, but an important part of self-respect. This is well recognized by psychologists and psychiatrists, and skin and hair care is often an important adjunctive treatment in depressive states.

These, then, are some of the reasons for writing this book. Myths and inaccuracies on skin care, skin disease, and what cosmetics can do for the skin are common, and it can be difficult for the average man, or more likely, woman, in the street to sort out fact from fiction. I hope that this book will help to do this.

I would like to thank Gordon Munro for drawing the illustrations on pp. 2, 3, and 81.

Preface

I am particularly grateful to Una Syme for her rapid and efficient typing and word processing skills, and also to my editor at OUP for her friendly advice and encouragement.

R.M.M.

Glasgow
March 1992

Contents

Contents

Contents

1.

Essential facts about the skin

This chapter is some basic facts about the skin—its composition, how it looks under the microscope, and how it works—and will make the medical terms used in the rest of the book understandable. It is probably the heaviest reading in the book and initially you may wish to turn straight to the area that is of most interest to you. If you do this, remember that terms that may be unclear are explained here.

COMPOSITION OF THE SKIN

Skin is composed of three main parts:

(1) the **epidermis**, or outer layer;
(2) the **dermis**, or deeper layer;
(3) the **skin appendages**—structures that pass through the dermis and epidermis and come into contact with the outside world on the surface. These are the hairs, the sweat glands, and other more specialized glands.

Figure 1 shows the relation between the epidermis, the underlying dermis, the hair roots, and other skin appendages that are situated in the dermis but which pass through the epidermis to the outside world. Between the epidermis and the dermis is a very specialized layer that acts like glue—'sticking' the epidermis and dermis together; this is the **basement membrane**.

THE EPIDERMIS

The basic living units of the body are the **cells**. Specialized cells are found in most parts of the body including the brain, the liver, the lungs, and the skin. A cell is composed of a central power house— the nucleus—that tells it what to do. The nucleus is surrounded by

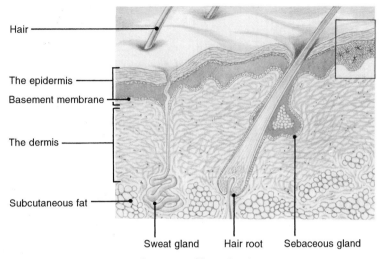

Hair

The epidermis

Basement membrane

The dermis

Subcutaneous fat

Sweat gland   Hair root   Sebaceous gland

Figure 1   An outline map of how the skin is constructed.

material called **cytoplasm**, which is enclosed by the **cell membrane**. The individual cells in the epidermis are very closely packed, with space between them—like a well-built brick wall—so that the membrane of one cell is in close contact with that of the adjacent cells.

The epidermis is composed of many individual cells of three types:

(1) keratinocytes;
(2) melanocytes;
(3) Langerhans cells.

Keratinocytes

The bulk of the epidermis is made up of **keratinocytes**. These cells are responsible for producing the outer surface layer of the epidermis—the cornified layer, sometimes referred to in older medical textbooks as the stratum corneum. Viewed down the microscope, the epidermis looks somewhat like a brick wall, with the keratinocytes forming most of the bricks and the other two types of cell— the melanocytes and the Langerhans cells—scattered here and there, mainly in the lower part of the epidermis (see Figure 2).

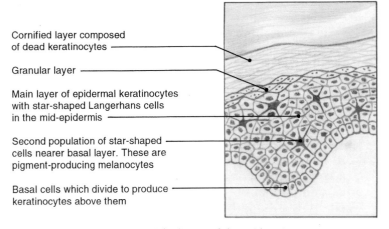

Cornified layer composed
of dead keratinocytes

Granular layer

Main layer of epidermal keratinocytes
with star-shaped Langerhans cells
in the mid-epidermis

Second population of star-shaped
cells nearer basal layer. These are
pigment-producing melanocytes

Basal cells which divide to produce
keratinocytes above them

Figure 2   The layers of the epidermis.

Melanocytes

The cells in the epidermis responsible for skin colour are the **melanocytes**. About one cell in every ten in the lowest layer of the epidermis is a melanocyte and is responsible for producing the pigment, called melanin, that gives rise to an individual's skin colour. The melanocytes are stimulated to activity by exposure to sunlight. Melanocytes in darker-skinned individuals are more active and produce larger quantities of pigment than those in fairer-skinned people. Those born with a genetically dark skin do not have more melanocytes than Caucasians: they simply have melanocytes that produce pigment more rapidly and in rather larger granules to spread around the surrounding keratinocytes.

Melanocytes are responsible for protecting the other cells of the skin against the damaging effects of sunlight. If white skin is exposed to strong sunlight, the melanocytes (which are found mostly in the lower layers of the epidermis) are stimulated to produce the protective melanin pigment. This brown pigmentation is responsible for the deepening skin colour of a suntan, and is a sign that the epidermis has been mildly damaged and that the melanocyte is trying to produce a shield of protective pigment over the keratinocyte nuclei. The melanocyte does this first, by making the melanin pigment itself, and then by injecting the little particles or granules of melanin into the cytoplasm of the adjacent keratino-cyte. The granules of melanin cluster together immediately above the keratinocyte nuclei and absorb some of the sun's rays when they pass through the upper layers of the epidermis, thus protecting the nuclei of the basal layer keratinocytes. Without this protection, greater damage would be done to the keratinocyte nucleus—damage that could be the first step in the development of a skin cancer. This will be discussed in much more detail in Chapter 7.

Just as the leopard in Rudyard Kipling's *Just So* stories cannot change its spots, so the skin cannot change the way it reacts to sunlight. Some people, especially those with some Southern European ancestry, and dark hair, and dark eyes, will rapidly develop a deep suntan if they are out-of-doors in sunny weather. However, in Northern Europe and many northern US states the more common type of skin is pale with freckles and pale brown or red hair and blue eyes. These people tend to go pink and peel in the sun and a tan, if it is acquired at all, is the end result of a slow and often painful process.

Langerhans cells

The third main type of cell in the epidermis is the **Langerhans cell**. These cells form only 2–4 per cent of the cells in the epidermis; they sit in the mid-zone of the epidermis, looking rather like large octopi. They have a central body and many 'tentacles', long processes extending out, just like the tentacles of an octopus, which reach out between and around the surrounding keratinocytes.

The Langerhans cells are thought to be important in the body's immune defences. Foreign material, for example tiny particles of nickel from a watch-strap or an ear-ring, passing through the epidermis from the outside, usually come into contact with the long 'tentacles' of the Langerhans cells. The particles stick to the 'tentacles' and are carried by the cell to other parts of the body. Langerhans cells can move from the epidermis through the base-ment membrane, into the dermis, and then via the small lymphatic vessels that drain fluid from the skin to the lymph glands or lymph nodes, which are concentrated in the groin, neck, and armpits. It is in the lymph nodes that the absorbed foreign material is processed; it is then eliminated from the body, without our ever being aware of it, although for a few unfortunate people this processing results in the development of allergic contact dermatitis (see p. 41) and, the next time the material in question is handled, an irritating rash develops.

For the skin to operate successfully, the epidermis and the dermis must stick together, and not slide over each other. Joining the epidermis and dermis is a complex structure—the **basement membrane**. This membrane itself has many different layers and is responsible for literally holding the skin together. If individual layers in the basement membrane are faulty, the epidermis and the dermis become separated and body fluids move into the space created, causing a blister. This can happen either as an inborn problem—as a rare group of diseases in young babies called **epidermolysis bullosa**—or as a disease that develops in older patients later in life—**bullous pemphigoid.**

THE DERMIS

The deepest layer of the skin—the one on which the keratinocytes rest—is the **dermis**. Using the brick wall analogy, the dermis is the solid ground on which the wall is built. There are fewer cells in the dermis than in the epidermis, and they are surrounded by fibres of a material called **collagen**, which hold the dermis, and the epidermis on top of it, to the rest of the body by tiny threads (see Figure 2). The dermis also contains many elastic fibres that make the skin supple, so that it stretches when we move, and can then move back into place.

The cells in the dermis are not quite as specialized as the keratinocytes of the epidermis. Many of them are **fibroblasts**, which are also found in many other parts of the body. These cells make the collagen that surrounds them and are particularly important when the skin is cut or wounded, when they quickly produce more collagen. Healing is further facilitated by the keratinocytes in the epidermis, which move in to fill the gap. This process of wound healing goes on underneath the scab that forms after injury.

The dermis is essential for the health and well-being of the overlying epidermal cells. The nutritional and energy requirements of the epidermis are supplied through the small blood vessels found in the dermis. Also in the dermis are the specialized nerves that make the skin an important sensory organ through which we feel touch, pain, heat, and cold. A sense of pain is an essential protection against injury, for example from burns.

The dermis can also synthesize vitamin D after exposure to sunlight. In countries where the dietary intake of vitamin D is low, this form of vitamin D synthesis can be important in ensuring that people have adequate levels of the vitamin, although individuals on a normal western diet, which contains ample vitamin D, usually have very little need for this sunlight-induced vitamin D synthesis.

THE SKIN APPENDANGES

The skin appendages are the hair follicle, the sebaceous or grease-producing glands, the sweat glands (eccrine and apocrine glands), and the nails.

Hair

Hair is obviously most numerous on the scalp, but there are also fine hairs on other body sites. Scalp hair is referred to as **terminal** or **coarse hair** and fine body hair found, for example, on the forearm, as **vellous hair**.

Hair is composed of modified keratinocytes. The very deepest part of the hair root—the **papilla**—is developed from the deepest part of the skin—the dermis—but most of the hair shaft develops from an ingrowth into the dermis of the epidermal keratinocytes before birth. These keratinocytes grow down and develop into the complicated structure that is the hair. As with the epidermis, the only part of the hair that is actually living is the deepest root area—all the hair seen above the skin surface is composed of dead, non-dividing cells.

Hair follicles go through a slow, programmed pattern of growth and replacement. Over a period of about 2 years individual hair follicles (roots) go through a cycle of rapid growth, rest, then the hair is shed. This pattern of programmed replacement of hair is usually random over the scalp, and therefore at any one time no obvious areas of hair loss are seen on healthy scalps in children or women, although some men do experience permanent loss of scalp hair as they get older. Fewer hairs are lost during pregnancy, when the hair on the head can seem temporarily thicker. After delivery of the child, however, this advantage is lost and more hair goes into the resting or shedding phase. The scalp hair therefore becomes temporarily thinner, returning to its regular cycle about 9 months after the birth.

The sebaceous or grease-producing glands

The sebaceous glands produce a thick, greasy liquid—**sebum**—which lubricates the skin and helps keep it smooth and waterproof. These glands are attached to the part of the hair shaft growing out from the hair root in the dermis towards the epidermis (see Figure 1). Sebaceous glands are found in large numbers on the face, upper back, and chest; they are less numerous on other body sites. Their ability to secrete sebum is partly controlled by hormones circulating in the bloodstream. They may be temporarily large for the first day or two after birth due to the effect of hormones from the mother's blood on the glands of the newborn baby. However, after this they are small and inactive throughout childhood, until the start of puberty at the age of 10–13 years. At puberty the child's own hormones stir the glands into activity and for the next few years these glands are usually very active—and sometimes over active, causing acne (see Chapter 4).

The sweat glands

There are two types of sweat glands in the skin—the **eccrine** sweat glands, and the **apocrine** sweat glands.

Eccrine glands

The eccrine glands are found all over the body. They make and secrete perspiration, which is one of the body's ways of losing excess heat. Even when we are not visibly perspiring, these glands are continually allowing a little fluid to escape from the body. This insensible fluid loss is greater in a dry, low-humidity environment, such as an aeroplane or a well-heated house, because the dry atmosphere is literally sucking moisture out of the skin. Extra fluid replacement with water or other non-alcoholic drinks is needed in such situations.

Fluid loss and control of body temperature through the sweat glands is very important in hot, humid, tropical environments. A few unlucky people are born with small numbers of eccrine sweat glands that do not function well. Such people can be uncomfortable and unwell in a tropical country, and may even get serious heatstroke. This happened to the character played by Shirley Eaton in the James Bond film *Goldfinger*. The character was coated all over with gold leaf or gold paint and because there was no connection between her skin and the air, no fluid or heat could escape through her pores or from her sweat glands, and her body temperature rose fatally. This is a real possibility, not a film-maker's fantasy.

Apocrine glands

The second type of sweat gland—the apocrine sweat glands—are found almost exclusively in the armpit and secrete a material much thicker than ordinary perspiration. They work particularly when we are nervous or stressed, and their secretion has a characteristic odour, which is regarded as undesirable in most cultures and that can be removed by the use of a deodorant. Alternatively, the activity of the apocrine glands can be temporarily turned off by an antiperspirant.

The nails

Like the hair, nails consist of modified epidermal keratinocytes. Here again, before birth there is an ingrowth of the epidermis, in this case growing to form a nail plate on which the hard nail structure is formed. As with hair, the outer cells composing the nail are dead. Nowadays, nails have relatively minor function, for example for picking up pins and other small objects, but clearly in evolution the presence of nails or claws was extremely useful in climbing trees, for gathering food, and for personal grooming. In monkeys, and particularly chimpanzees, the firm structure of a nail at the end of the fingers is very important for many everyday functions. As humans evolved, we learned to use tools as a substitute for our fingernails.

HOW THE SKIN WORKS

The epidermis is constantly replacing itself. Snakes literally shed their whole skin and emerge with a bright new skin, leaving the wrinkled cast behind. Human skin renewal is not as dramatic but, over a period of about 4 weeks, we also shed our entire skin surface.

The cells in the epidermis are living, and all living cells divide into two daughter cells. In normal skin this process of cell division takes place only in the deepest layer of the epidermis—the **basal layer**. When it happens, one of the daughter keratinocytes remains in the basal layer, and will in time divide again.

The second keratinocyte moves upwards through the epidermis, slowly working its way from the the basal layer to the uppermost layer of keratinocytes. This cell will not divide again in the course of its journey through the epidermis, and is programmed to self-destruct and die. During its passage through the epidermis it changes shape. In the lower layers it is a rather square cell with a large round nucleus and a small amount of surrounding cytoplasm. As it moves up through the epidermis it first becomes larger and then, about two-thirds of the way through the epidermis, a dramatic change takes place—the keratinocyte becomes much flatter and the nucleus breaks up to form many small granules in the cytoplasm. Above the area where this happens the keratinocytes 'ghosts' are totally dead and have no nucleus. This outermost layer—the **cornified layer** of the skin—can be seen without a microscope as fine scaling from the skin surface. This scaling is seen more frequently in those with dry skin, or after an injury such as mild sunburn. Cosmetics containing a mild abrasive ('scrubs') are designed to remove this outer dead layer of skin cells and make the skin look fresher because the underlying, pinker, living cells are brought nearer to the skin surface. If the sticky surface of transparent tape is repeatedly stuck on and then removed from the same area of skin it is possible to remove a large number of these superficial or dead cells from the epidermis and leave a pink, rather tender, glistening layer of living cells underneath.

In normal skin the entire process of keratinocytes dividing, moving from the basal layer area of the epidermis to the outer layer, and being shed into the surrounding environment takes about 28 days.

THE FUNCTIONS OF THE SKIN

The Table overleaf gives a list of the various tasks the skin carries out, and the parts of the skin responsible for these tasks.

The skin is responsible for protecting the contents of the body from the outside world, and for holding them together.

Table 1   The tasks of the skin

Tasks	Part of skin responsible
Holding the body contents together	Epidermis and keratinocytes
Waterproofing	Keratinocytes and lipids
Protection from sunlight	Epidermal melanocytes
Recognition of 'non-self' material entering through the epidermis	Langerhans' cells in epidermis
Control of body temperature	Dermal blood vessels
Production of pain to warn of damage	Pain-sensitive nerve endings in upper dermis
Protection from infection	Whole epidermis and lipids

FLUID LOSS

As we have seen, the skin also has a role in controlling fluid loss from the body by perspiration, and in the temperature control of the body. After exercise, when the skin becomes flushed and warm, the blood vessels in the skin expand and fill up, so heat is lost from the blood through the skin.

Such fluid loss also results in the loss of some body salts. This means that to restore the body's fluid balance it is necessary not only to drink water, but also to take in some salts or electrolytes. In a cool climate, such as the UK, this can be done as part of the normal diet, but at times of intense exercise, or in a tropical climate, some extra table salt is a good idea. The agonizing muscle cramps that can affect some people during exercise or in hot situations is a sign that the body is short of salt, some of which will have been lost through the skin.

INFECTION

The skin protects us against many types of infection by both bacteria and viruses. If the surface of the epidermis is broken in any way it is very much easier for infection to set in and develop.

THE RELATIONSHIP BETWEEN THE SKIN AND THE REST OF THE BODY

It is important to realize that the skin is not an isolated structure detached from the rest of the body, but that it has excellent lines of communication through the bloodstream to the large blood vessels that take bloodborne substances to the heart, lungs, and other parts of the body. Therefore, events on the skin affect other parts of the body and can be associated with problems and at times, even illness can be associated with other parts of the body, such as the lungs or lymph glands. For example, in the acute stages of some skin diseases, the superficial blood vessels in the skin are permanently dilated, so the amount of blood passing through the skin is greatly increased. In time the heart can become strained by the additional work of pumping this extra blood through the skin, and mild heart failure can result.

The layers of the skin are continuous with the linings of the inner cavities of the body—the **mucous membranes**. The margin between skin and mucous membrane can easily be seen, for example, on the inner surface of the lip and on the lower eyelid at the line of the eyelashes. Often when the skin is involved in a disease or abnormality, the mucous membranes are also involved, which is why the doctors may want to look inside the mouth if there is a problem or a rash elsewhere on the body.

SKIN GRAFTS

The cells in both the epidermis and dermis are relatively specific to any one person and transplanting skin between different people is even more difficult than performing kidney or heart transplants. Cells in the epidermis and the dermis carry what is best thought of as a code. This code is called the **human leucocyte antigen** or HLA system, and different markers are found on the cell surfaces in different code combinations. It is very rare for two people, other than identical twins, to have a perfect match of HLA systems.

At the present time there is great interest in the importance of these specific markers in the skin. It is hoped that, over the next decade, we will come to understand these HLA antigens better and be able to manipulate, and possibly change, them on skin grown in the test tube. Once this is possible it may become very much easier to treat people with severe burns. At present, even if such individuals have a skin graft from a non-identical twin, the graft, although it acts as a very good dressing, is eventually rejected. If it becomes possible to transfer skin from one individual to another, and for that skin to grow in a normal healthy way, some of the serious scarring, skin damage and even death caused by severe burns could be prevented.

LIMITATIONS OF THE SKIN

The skin cannot permanently change its colour, or the way that it reacts to sunlight. In western countries, many white-skinned people persist in trying to keep their skins permanently browner than nature intended, by sunbathing in summer, and by the use of sun-beds in winter. This will cause early ageing of the skin and can, in time, make skin cancer more likely.

In contrast, in countries where a white skin is more desirable, such as South Africa, bleaching creams may be used in an attempt to lighten the skin. These creams can be absorbed through the skin and deposited in the cartilage found deep under the skin, where they may cause a very disfiguring condition called **ochronosis**. This is a disfiguring slate-grey colour that affects the soft bones or cartilage of the nose and cheeks due to deposition of dark pigments.

While the skin is very good at repairing superficial epidermal damage with no residual scar, if the dermis is damaged a scar of some type is inevitable. The structure of the epidermis, and the fact that it is continually renewing itself, means that repair is easy and relatively rapid. The epidermis heals very rapidly when we are young, and in children who frequently graze their skin, causing breaks in the epidermis, the damage may be totally repaired in a few days, while the same type of damage on the leg of their grandmother may take weeks to heal. This is one of the effects of ageing on the skin—it renews itself more slowly as we get older. However, if the skin is damaged down to the level of the dermis there will be a scar once healing is completed. Most surgical procedures to the skin involve the dermis and therefore must cause a scar—a fact that should be remembered if a mole or birthmark is to be removed for cosmetic rather than medical reasons. If the birthmark is very small and relatively inconspicuous, the scar left after removal could be more of a cosmetic inconvenience than the original blemish.

AGEING

As we grow older our skin gradually becomes drier. As we will see in Chapter 6, the sebaceous glands, which produce a lot, but not all, of the greasy or oily material that lubricates our skin, are very active in the teenage years but become less active with age. Women who use cosmetics will notice that, although in their teens and twenties they found preparations labelled as suitable for greasy skin most satisfactory, 20 years later preparations for dry skin seem to suit them better. This is because of the slowing down of the output of the sebaceous glands.

In fact, the explanation for differing skin types is even more complicated than this, as oily or greasy material is also produced by the epidermal keratinocytes, and contributes to the protective waterproofing of the skin and to its suppleness. In addition, however, this oily or lipid material from the sebaceous glands and keratinocytes also helps the body retain water by preventing evaporation of water from the skin surface. So both lipids and water, acting together, are important in preventing skin from drying out. Moisturizing creams can therefore be very light-acting, mainly by improving water retention, or much heavier, for example night creams, which mainly contain oils and heavy emollients. The importance of cosmetics is discussed further in Chapter 9.

2.

Infants and toddlers

The next few chapters will look at the way the skin behaves at different stages in our lives. In many ways, the skin has several ages, and different skin problems are more or less common at different ages. It is therefore sensible to look at skin problems and characteristics according to age.

THE FIRST FEW WEEKS

At birth a baby usually has smooth, perfect skin. The skin of many babies, particularly those that are a little overdue, may peel a little in the first week of life. This is most often seen on the hands and feet, and is perfectly normal and nothing to worry about. Most babies have fine downy scalp hair at birth, but some have a thick growth of dark hair. Babies who are born with thick dark hair very often shed this first growth of hair within the first month of life and temporarily look rather bald. Once again, this is nothing to worry about; the baby's hair will grow normally from then on.

Many new mothers are worried about the appearance of their infant's finger-nails and toe-nails, which, particularly those of the fifth fingers and toes, may appear rather small and curved. These will straighten out naturally during the first 6 months of life. Action should be taken only if the baby is older than this and is clearly having discomfort with a finger- or toe-nail digging into the surrounding flesh.

One of the common observations within a few days of birth is that the newborn baby has a crop of little white or yellow papules around the nose and cheeks. This is due to temporary activity of the sebaceous or grease-producing glands. These grease-producing glands, which are discussed in much more detail in Chapter 1 (p. 7) are temporarily stimulated into activity by the mother's hormones, some of which are still circulating in the baby's blood. These hormones cause a brief burst of activity in the baby's sebaceous glands and make them look large and very visible for a few days. These papules normally disappear in the first week or two of life as the mother's hormones disappear from the baby's blood. These little glands on the face then remain present but inactive until the child is aged 10–12 years, when once again they are stimulated into activity, this time by the child's own hormonal activity.

Very occasionally, the grease-producing or sebaceous glands on the faces of newborn babies do not become totally inactive after the first 2 weeks of life, and a mild form of acne develops. This can easily be treated and controlled and is almost always seen in male rather than in female babies.

TEMPERATURE CONTROL

A newborn baby has a very large surface area of skin relative to its height and weight, and it is therefore easy for it to lose a lot of heat across its skin surface. This can happen very rapidly and is the reason why small infants should be protected from sudden chilling and should be wrapped quickly in a warm, dry towel after bathing.

The opposite situation can also develop, and it is not at all uncommon for new mothers to be so anxious to prevent their newborn infant from being cold that they over-protect it. In the winter months, a new baby may be wrapped in a woollen vest and woollen outer garments with several blankets on top, and nursed in a well-insulated pram, cot or carry-cot in a centrally heated room. The baby's small sweat glands will struggle to control the overheating. The infant's sweat glands can usually cope with this, but sometimes they are asked to do more work than they are yet capable of and the infant may develop a rash, usually on the stomach and back. This rash is composed of small raised red bumps and is referred to as **prickly heat**. Mothers who have brought up babies in the tropics will know very well what this looks like because it is difficult to avoid in a hot, humid tropical environment. Another place where prickly heat is quite commonly seen is in the hot and humid atmosphere of the special care nursery for very premature babies. Prickly heat is easily prevented by removing a layer or two of clothing from the baby or by reducing the temperature in the room where he or she sleeps. A light dusting of a normal baby powder or an application of calamine lotion will make the infant more comfortable while the rash subsides. In general, cotton, rather than wool, next to the skin is best, both to reduce minor irritation and to prevent prickly heat.

BATH-TIME

For a newborn baby, bath-time is not usually an occasion when vigorous cleaning of the skin is needed. The napkin area is an obvious exception and will be discussed next. In a year or two, when the child is an active toddler, this situation will change dramatically! For a newborn baby, a bath is a social occasion, and should be enjoyable for both parent and child, a time when they get to know each other and for the baby to gain a little confidence as he or she is handled, and to learn to splash in water and to enjoy it. The bath should be at a moderate temperature and the baby can be washed with a normal brand of soap, a special infant soap, or one of the special infant bathing lotions that are widely available. Most babies' skin reacts perfectly well to the use of a mild, non-perfumed soap, which must, of course, be kept away from the eyes. It is important to rinse all soap off thoroughly because traces of soap left on the skin will cause some drying of the skin and may make the baby uncomfortable. After the bath, and after the skin has been patted dry, a small quantity of talcum power may be dusted in the skin creases, and this will probably make the infant feel more comfortable. Otherwise, no special care is required for normal infant skin in the first few months of life.

CARE OF THE SKIN OF THE NAPKIN AREA

Over the first 2 years of life the skin of the napkin area is put to a very harsh test. Until the baby learns to control both bladder and bowel, the delicate skin of the newborn child is continuously subjected to the drying and irritating effects of urine and bowel movements. At this stage of life, the skin in this area is asked to tolerate more than it will ever be required to tolerate again until, perhaps the complications of extreme old age.

The general principle of care of the napkin area is to keep it dry but with a protective film of lubricating cream to protect the skin from urine. This involves the sensible choice and regular changing of napkins, and also the use as required of appropriate nappy creams and ointments—partly to act as a waterproofing agent to protect the skin from the damaging effects of urine, and partly to replace the grease on the skin surface that is constantly being removed by the effects of urine and of cleansing the area.

The choice of napkins for a new baby will depend on many things. Some mothers have strong views about the use of cloth or of disposable napkins, and this may depend on the availability of laundry, the availability of appropriate facilities for disposal of napkins, cost, concern for the environment and other factors. Generally speaking, there are no specific dermatological reasons for selecting cloth or disposable napkins, provided that if cloth napkins are chosen they are appropriately laundered to remove all trace of urine and other material. Cloth napkins are best dried out-of-doors on a washing-line, as the action of fresh air and sunshine will freshen them, make them soft, and also help destroy some of the bacteria that may not have been entirely removed during the washing and rinsing process. In the winter months, however, this is not always practical.

Although disposable napkins initially seem relatively expensive compared to cloth napkins, the newer napkins, which claim to be 'superabsorbent' do, in many cases, justify this claim. Scientific studies comparing the amount of fluid that can be absorbed and removed from the skin surface by cloth and by disposable napkins show that some of the newer superabsorbent napkins work very well indeed. In addition, the surface of some superabsorbent napkins removes moisture from the skin and does not allow it to seep back in, provided that the napkin is changed relatively frequently. Thus, if the baby has problems with nappy rash, a temporary or even permanent investment in these superbrands is worth considering.

To prevent problems with napkin rash and irritation in this area, it is important to change the napkins regularly. There are no hard and fast rules about how often this should be and the general advice is that when the napkin is wet it should be changed. Mothers vary as to whether or not they wish to use a napkin cream regularly and there are a variety of preparations on the market, all of which are quite satisfactory. Most of these are ointments that act as a barrier between the skin and the urine. They have a mild waterproofing effect on the skin surface and will usually make the baby more comfortable. They are particularly useful at night, when it is likely that the baby will have to lie longer in a damp napkin than would be the case during the day. There are many proprietary napkin creams available, several based on zinc and castor oil. They are safe, soothing, and can be used in large quantities on the napkin area as required. It is important to remove all traces of urine or bowel movement from the child's skin before these creams are applied. This can be done either by the use of ready-moistened tissues, dampened cotton wool, or by soap and water and gentle drying with a towel. Creams and ointments containing steroids or hydro-cortisone should *not* be used as a regular napkin cream and are for short-term use only, and then only under the supervision of the family doctor.

If, despite care, mild napkin rash does develop, one of the best methods of curing it before it becomes a stubborn problem is to keep the child in a warmer than average room for a few days and to allow him or her to lie with the lower half of the body uncovered and a frequently changed napkin underneath. Napkin rash is due to a combination of the damp environment caused by urine and the interaction between urine and bowel movement, which allows bacteria found in the product of the digestive tract to break down and irritate the skin. The fresh air treatment does not allow urine to remain in contact with the skin for any length of time and thus prevents the breakdown and irritation that causes napkin rash. This treatment will produce a lot of extra washing for a few days, but is usually very worthwhile.

MINOR PROBLEMS AROUND THE TIME OF BIRTH

A small number of babies have minor skin abnormalities at birth. If these are on the face they often cause considerable distress to the parents, although the baby is otherwise perfectly healthy and is eating and sleeping well. Similar problems on other parts of the body may not cause nearly so much concern to the parents. Nevertheless, if there are any abnormalities or unusual features on a baby's skin, the family doctor should be consulted as to whether any special care or attention is necessary. A number of minor blemishes are not actually visible at birth but are first seen at the age of 2–4 weeks. These will therefore not have been seen by the midwife or nurses involved with the delivery of the baby, nor when the baby was checked prior to leaving the hospital.

BIRTHMARKS

The word birthmark describes an abnormality either of the skin's blood vessels or of the pigment-producing melanocyte cells in the skin. They are usually seen at birth but may appear within the first week or two of life.

Angiomas

The most common type of birthmark is an abnormality of the blood vessels. These abnormalities—**angiomas**— are very common and are present in as many as one baby in ten. Quite a large number of these angiomas first appear at the age of about 1 week. Thus, the new mother, shortly after she has taken her baby home, notices a small red mark that she is fairly sure was not present at birth. A common worry is that the mark has appeared because the baby's skin has been damaged, perhaps by a finger-nail or by a small burn. This is not so; the angioma develops on skin that has not been damaged in any way.

The most common type of angioma is a **cavernous angioma**, sometimes referred to as a strawberry naevus because the surface of the birthmark resembles a strawberry. This type of angioma begins as a small pinkish area anywhere on the skin surface, but most commonly on the head and neck. During the first 6 months or so of the baby's life these birthmarks tend to grow quite rapidly and become raised above the skin surface. Because of this, parents can be very distressed and concerned that their baby is going to be left with a disfiguring birthmark for the rest of its life. However, these strawberry marks rarely grow for longer than 6 months, when they stop growing and will generally remain static for another 6 months or so. After this time they will slowly shrink and become very much paler.

Thus, by the time the baby is aged around 2, a birthmark that was very obvious at 6 months is hardly visible at all and may only be seen as an area of paler, slightly wrinkled skin. There is no

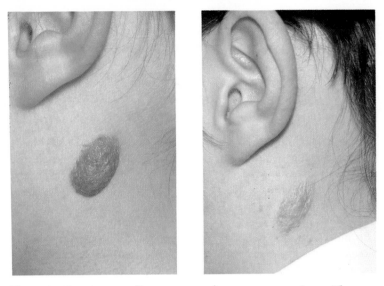

Figure 3 Spontaneous disappearance of a cavernous angioma. The same child is illustrated aged 6 months (left) and then at 9 years (right). There has been no treatment of this angioma.

surgical or dermatological treatment that will give as good a final cosmetic result on the child's skin as letting nature take its course. The illustrations in Figure 3 show just how true this is. Most children with these angiomas require no treatment at all, although some parents may be happier if the child is seen every 6 months or so by a specialist, just to make sure that the angioma is shrinking naturally as expected in the way described above. Sometimes, when a large strawberry naevus has finished shrinking, a small plastic surgery operation is needed to remove loose skin, but this is the exception rather than the rule.

When the strawberry mark is at its most obvious, between the ages of around 6 months and a year, it can be rather fragile, and bleeding from these birthmarks at this stage is not uncommon. This may be because the child has scratched the lesion or because it is in the napkin area and is constantly irritated. If vigorous bleeding occurs, and this is uncommon, gentle pressure on the area with a cotton wool ball wil help to stop it fairly quickly. The blood vessels in these angiomas are fairly small and there is absolutely no risk of serious bleeding. One of the good results of such bleeding, if it

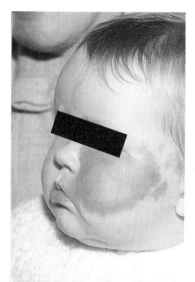

Figure 4 Capillary naevus. Unlike the angioma in Figure 3, this mark will not become less obvious with age unless it is treated.

does take place, is that very often the natural shrinkage of the birthmark is speeded up as a result of the damage to the blood vessels.

Stork marks or capillary naevi

A second type of birthmark arising from blood vessels is called the stork mark or **capillary naevus**. This may be present in a very mild form on the nape of the neck or on the skin of the face between the eyes. A slightly more extensive form may be seen covering part of one cheek or the chin or forehead (Figure 4). These capillary naevi are frequently present at birth, and do not tend to grow above the level of the skin surface like the strawberry naevus. The surface of the child's skin is smooth and regular, like the surface of the other cheek, but the colour is different and the cheek is permanently pink, becoming a darker shade of red if the child is very hot or distressed and crying. These capillary naevi do not tend to shrink spontaneously and without treatment they will remain unchanged. Until recently the best treatment for such vascular naevi was to provide a cosmetic cover-up cream, which can be used by either sex and which completely hides the birthmark. This has been quite satisfactory for most people, but involves spending 10 minutes or so each morning applying the cream.

Lasers and birthmarks

Exciting developments using laser therapy for correcting the blood vessel abnormality in these capillary naevi are now taking place. Laser treatment involves the use of a specialized type of light delivered at a very high energy along a tube with a diameter of only a few millimetres. There are many different types of laser. At present, the tunable dye is most promising for the treatment of angiomas. The laser beam destroys the small blood vessels that give rise to the unusual colour in capillary naevi. Because of the small size of the laser beam, laser treatment involves many sessions, at each of which only a small area of skin can be treated. It is important to treat each area only once, to avoid scarring, and it is therefore essential for the patient to lie very still, and for this reason it may be necessary to use a general anaesthetic. At the present time laser treatment for vascular birthmarks is being introduced in a small number of National Health Service hospitals in the UK, although it is more widely available in North America. Treatment is time-consuming for both doctor and patient, but the results are encouraging. It is highly likely that over the next few years this form of treatment will become more widely available, and the need for camouflage cover treatment will become less.

Congenital melanocytic naevi or moles

The other main group of birthmarks arises from the melanocytes. Almost everyone has small, totally benign, non-worrying moles or naevi on the skin. These are small collections of brown pigment-producing melanocytes, which are usually found in the lower layer of the epidermis and in the dermis. Most young adults have around 20 to 30 such moles, usually between 2 and 4 mm in diameter, and the great majority of these first appear between the ages of 12 and 20 years. However, about one baby in a hundred is born with a congenital melanocytic naevus, or mole. This type of birthmark is usually present at birth, although, as with the blood vessel birthmarks, a small proportion first appear between the ages of 1 and 4 weeks. They are usually seen as a faint brown mark on any part of the body and may vary in size from about 1 cm in diameter to covering quite a large area of skin. Over the first few months of the baby's life these moles often become very much darker and occasionally there is a fine growth of downy hair.

Babies born to darker-skinned parents frequently have a bluish mark present over the lower back area at birth. This is quite a normal finding in Asian babies, and is not associated with unusual hair growth; it is sometimes called a Mongolian spot. It usually becomes paler as the child grows and in time will disappear almost completely.

Congenital melanocytic naevi or brown moles present at birth do not need any immediate treatment unless they start to grow or change in any way. If a baby has a mole of this type it is advisable to ask the family doctor for referral to a dermatological specialist to decide whether or not any special supervision is needed. A common practice in the case of these moles is to take one or two close-up photographs with a ruler or other scale beside the mole so that any change can be quickly noticed. Other than this, no special treatment is usually required.

Moles on the face may result in the child being teased when they start nursery school, and some parents wish the moles removed because of this. Remember that there is no way to remove a mole without leaving a scar, and sometimes the scar can cause almost as much distress as the mole. There are no medical reasons for removing congenital brown moles in early childhood unless they show signs of growth or other change.

There is at the present time no one established treatment pattern for these congenital moles, but many specialists believe that removing the moles in later childhood, when the child is aged between 9 and 12 and can cooperate with a local anaesthetic, is a good policy. This is because there is a very slight risk that a mole could become malignant and cancerous in later life. It must be emphasized that this is a low risk and that, as the type of cancer involved very, very rarely affects children, it is perfectly safe to delay the removal of these moles until the child is approaching puberty. The very slight risk of a small congenital naevus becoming malignant probably does not justify a general anaesthetic, which of course also carries a slight risk. It is therefore better to wait until the child has reached an age when they understand what is involved, and can cooperate with a local anaesthetic.

Babies affected by the very rare giant congenital naevus will be referred to a specialist centre, and the possible approaches to removing some or all of the naevus will be explained to the parents by an expert, usually a plastic surgeon.

ECZEMA AND THE SMALL BABY

Eczema is an inflammation of the skin that causes the sensation of itch and makes the sufferer want to scratch. An alternative name for eczema is dermatitis—the two terms mean exactly the same thing and it is not uncommon for some doctors to use the term eczema to describe the problem in babies and dermatitis in older children and adults. The two types of eczema which can affect young babies are **seborrhoeic eczema** and **atopic eczema**.

SEBORRHOEIC ECZEMA

Seborrhoeic eczema is now relatively uncommon, although 30 years ago it was a common problem in the large childrens' hospitals in big cities. Nowadays, in these same cities it is comparatively rare, although we do not understand why the numbers of children with this type of eczema have fallen so strikingly.

Seborrhoeic eczema usually affects small babies when they are less than 3 months old. It can be recognized by the presence of fairly extensive scaling on the scalp. It is quite normal for many babies to have a slight scurf on the scalp, rather like excessive dandruff. This is sometimes referred to as cradle cap (Figure 5). In seborrhoeic eczema this cradle cap pattern is more extensive than usual and may even involve the forehead down to the eyebrows. In addition, the baby may have a red, scaly rash in the napkin area and under the arms. The napkin area rash will develop despite the parents' best efforts to keep the area clean and dry. Although seborrhoeic eczema is obviously distressing to parents, the striking thing as far as the baby is concerned is that they seem totally untroubled by the rash and eat well and sleep normally. Thus, seborrhoeic eczema does not appear to cause the baby much itch or other discomfort.

Treatment
Seborrhoeic eczema is usually best treated by a small quantity of relatively mild topical steroid creams. These must be prescribed by

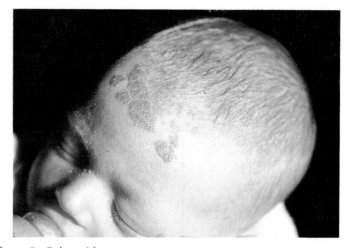

Figure 5 Baby with seborrhoeic eczema. Note scaly scalp and the fact that the baby seems in no discomfort.

a doctor and should be used exactly as prescribed. It is particularly important not to put stronger steroid creams on the facial skin, especially on small babies.

Seborrhoeic eczema generally clears up completely before the baby is 6 months old and is therefore only a temporary problem. At present there is no evidence to suggest that babies who have seborrhoeic eczema have other problems later in life.

ATOPIC ECZEMA

Atopic eczema is often a more severe and persistent type of eczema than the seborrhoeic type. It tends to run in families and may be associated with chest problems, including asthma and hay fever. In contrast to seborrhoeic eczema, babies with atopic eczema tend to look as if they are uncomfortable. Before their fingers are coordinated and they are able to scratch, a baby with atopic eczema will try to rub its cheek against the sheet or pillow, causing redness of the cheek's (Figure 6) skin. Once they can coordinate their fingers, small scratch marks will appear on the face, and when the entire skin is exposed at bath-time the baby may try to rub and scratch its tummy and other parts of the body. Babies with atopic eczema are

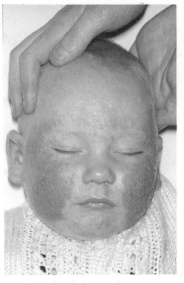

Figure 6 The red cheeks of a baby with atopic eczema who has been rubbing its cheek against bedding.

frequently a little irritable and tend to feed and sleep less well than other babies.

Most babies who develop atopic eczema do so between the age of 6 months and 1 year, and very often the cheeks and trunk are the areas most affected. Once he or she is a toddler the sites most affected change, and the arms in front of the elbow, the area behind the knees, and the ankle area become the most involved.

Atopic eczema is partly inherited. If one parent has a personal history of atopic eczema there is an increased risk of the child having the problem, and if both parents have a history of atopic eczema the risk is further increased.

Control and treatment of atopic eczema

Babies with atopic eczema often have a relatively dry skin. If you have a family history of atopic eczema, and you are concerned that your young baby may be developing this problem, it is a good policy to use a bath oil routinely. There are a large number of these available, some specially prepared for infant skin and others for all skins. Suitable preparations include Hydromol, Alpha Keri, and

Oilatum. It is a good idea to select a non-perfumed, lanolin-free bath oil, as both perfume and lanolin can give rise to problems with allergies. These allergies are much less common in children than in adults, but can still be a problem.

If a bath oil or additive is used in a baby's bath, remember that it makes both the bath and the baby very slippery. A small baby must be held very firmly if he or she is being bathed in such a bath, and an older toddler must be prevented from slipping and falling when getting into or out of the bath.

Most children with atopic eczema find a tepid bath with a bath oil added comforting and soothing, and the good that is being done by the emollient in the bath must not be undone by using a lot of soap. There are useful soap-free alternatives, one of the easiest and cheapest being emulsifying ointment BP, which can be obtained relatively inexpensively in a large pot from a chemist; no prescription is needed. This ointment contains no steroid, cortisone or other active ingredient and is a simple, greasy, cleansing ointment that will replace some of the essential oils that the child's skin lacks. It is a very effective cleanser and can be used in place of soap, both for general cleansing and in the napkin area. It is usually better not to use baby powder on a baby with a dry skin problem, especially if bath emollients and emulsifying ointment are being used. Baby powder is mildly drying and can become caked and matted if traces of the oil remain on the skin.

ECZEMA AND THE COLD SORE VIRUS

People with atopic eczema do not react to the cold sore virus in the normal way. Most of us, once we have been exposed to this virus (herpes simplex type 1) for the first time have a few small blisters inside our mouth. These are usually asymptomatic and therefore go undetected. As a result of this mild infection, we develop lifelong immunity. A few people do not develop this immunity and are prone to repeated attacks of small blisters, usually on the upper lip. Atopic eczema sufferers do not develop normal immunity and, if they come into contact with someone with a cold sore, may develop quite a severe and widespread infection. While this can be treated with very effective modern antiviral drugs, it is much better to avoid the problem in the first place. *It is therefore important that a baby with eczema should not come into contact with anyone who*

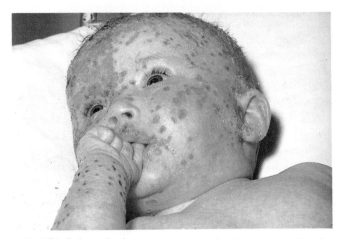

Figure 7   This baby, who has atopic eczema, has been exposed to the cold sore virus and now has eczema herpeticum. With prompt treatment this will heal without scarring, but it could have been prevented.

has the cold sore virus. Figure 7 shows a baby who has this problem. Information about protecting babies with atopy from the cold sore virus is not as widely available as it ought to be and should be given to all young mothers with babies with atopic eczema.

SUNSHINE

As will be emphasized repeatedly throughout this book, too much exposure to the sun damages the skin. It can cause drying, early wrinkles, an appearance of growing older before one's time, and can even, at the end of the day, predispose to skin cancer.

Most parents are happy to have their babies lie out-of-doors in sunny spring or summer weather, and fresh air is good for all of us. It is, however, very important to protect the skin of young babies— and indeed the skin of toddlers and older children—from excessive sun exposure. Small, white-skinned babies do not form a protective tan easily, and of course cannot move themselves out of direct sunlight into shade. It is surprisingly easy to cause redness and mild burning of a baby's skin if he or she is exposed to direct sunlight for even 20 minutes when the sun is at its height around midday.

For this reason, babies should be shaded from direct sunlight when they are out-of-doors. The pram can be parked under a tree, or a parasol can be used to protect the pram or push-chair when out walking. At the park or the beach, the rug or towel on which the baby sits should be spread under a tree or beach umbrella. These simple precautions are worth carrying out even in northern Europe and the northern American states because, during May, June, and July in particular, there are frequently bright, sunny days when the sun's rays can be very intense, although the air temperature is relatively cool.

Nowadays many parents take not only older children but also quite small babies on holiday to Mediterranean beaches. It is very important indeed to protect a baby's skin from the fierce Mediterranean sunlight. Small babies born in Mediterranean countries are well-protected from the sun by their parents, who are well aware of the strength of the Mediterranean sun and the damage it can do to an infant's skin. If you plan to take a small baby abroad to a sunny area on holiday, think carefully about the shade you will provide for the pram or carry-cot, and always make sure that this is parked where there is plenty of shade. Once your baby is able to sit up, he or she will thoroughly enjoy playing on the sand, but again make sure that this is under a parasol, and make sure he or she wears a large sun-bonnet or hat.

It is not only the skin that can suffer from strong sunlight: more serious problems, such as sun-stroke, can develop relatively easily. It is important, if you have a small baby in a hot, sunny environment, to be sure that he or she has plenty of extra fluid to drink, such as water or fruit juice, because a lot of body fluid will be lost through the skin.

A wide range of sunscreen preparations are now available and these will be discussed in greater detail in Chapter 7. Many sun-creams are made specifically for babies' skin. These are usually either complete sun-blocks or have a high skin protection factor (SPF). They are entirely suitable for the skin of small babies but should not be used to allow the child to spend a lot of time in direct sunlight. Use them sensibly to allow the child to spend time on the beach and in the water.

As with older children and adults, the skin of infants exposed to sunshine will tend to become rather dryer than usual. An after-sun cooling, soothing, emollient preparation at the end of the day is a good idea, and the addition of a bath oil or emollient to the bath will also help to prevent peeling and discomfort. It has been calculated that if the skin of children and teenagers were protected at all times from excessive sun exposure, then 78% of all skin cancers that develop later in life could be prevented. Over half of the sun exposure that a normal individual receives in their entire life takes place during childhood, so childhood is the time to learn sensible sun-exposure habits, and to learn about sun screens (see page 80).

3.

The younger child

Once toddlers are toilet-trained and running around independently, skin care for the next few years is relatively easy. Children between the ages of about 3 and 12 years are, of course, likely to do themselves a lot of minor damage, falling from tricycles and bicycles and in the course of sports and games on the playing field. Hygiene is therefore important and all cuts and grazes should be treated carefully, with gentle washing with a mild antiseptic and covering with an appropriate dry dressing until the area heals. Any non-healing area in a child or any sign of redness, infection and tenderness around the normal childhood grazes should arouse concern, and if the child is obviously uncomfortable an appointment to see the family doctor should be made without delay.

Once children are regularly in contact with others of their own age—in the playgroup, nursery school or primary school—they tend to develop a large number of minor infections. Many of these involve the skin and it is important to recognize these problems early, so that the child receives appropriate treatment, and so that the problem is not passed on to other children in the classroom or playgroup.

CHILDHOOD INFECTIOUS DISEASES AND THE SKIN

Common childhood infections that involve the child being generally unwell and that also involve the skin include:

(1) measles; due to the measles virus
(2) german measles; caused by the rubella virus
(3) chickenpox; caused by a pox virus
(4) scarlet fever; caused by the streptococcus.

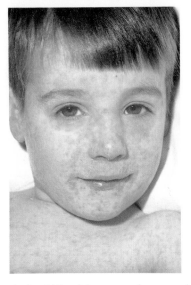

Figure 8   The typical red bloodshot eyes of a young boy with measles.

Children can be immunized against measles, German measles and scarlet fever and, unless there are very good reasons for the child not to receive these immunizations, it is a good policy to take advantage of all the immunizations routinely offered to you by your family doctor, health visitor or baby clinic. A doctor, paediatrician or health visitor will advise of any reasons for withholding or delaying any of these immunizations.

MEASLES

The child with early measles will be feverish, unwell, and listless. Very often the first signs of measles are seen around the eyes and the mouth. The child may have red eyes, a cough, a runny nose, and generally look miserable and feverish. (Figure 8).

Small white spots can be seen inside the mouth, on the inner surface of the cheeks. These spots are very often seen a day or two before the generalized measles rash develops and can be a helpful warning sign. At this stage measles cannot be prevented, but keeping the child warm and encouraging them to drink plenty of fluid can reduce their discomfort. They should also be kept away from other children, as this stage is the most infectious.

The measles rash usually begins as a blotchy red rash on the face and neck and then spreads down the body. Some parts of the rash, raised above the normal skin surface, can be felt as well as seen. As the rash begins to fade after 2 or 3 days, it often becomes a reddish brown colour, and the skin may start to peel.

GERMAN MEASLES (RUBELLA)

The rash of German measles is often only visible on the skin for about 24 hours. It is quite possible for a child to have German measles without being particularly unwell and even without the parents being aware of the infection. The German measles rash usually involves the face, chest, and back and is a very fine dusting of little red spots on the skin, rather like a dusting of Cayenne pepper. The lymph glands in the neck, just below the jaw, and also in the armpits and the groin, may be a little enlarged and tender. The child may complain of sore or stiff joints for a day or two.

German measles does not usually cause a lot of systemic upset in a young child, but if it is suspected it is essential to warn women with whom the child comes into contact and who might be in the early stages of pregnancy. German measles in the first 3 months of a pregnancy can damage the developing baby in the womb. For this reason it is very important that young girls know whether or not they have had German measles, as one attack usually confers life-long immunity. This is also the reason for giving small girls the German measles immunization and, if this has not been done in early childhood, it is important that teenage girls have a simple blood test to see whether or not they have had German measles and have therefore developed immunity to further attacks. If not, they should be immunized at this age to prevent any future tragedies.

CHICKENPOX

The rash of chickenpox is relatively easy to recognize. Fairly large, raised, palpable spots develop all over the child's body, but often most markedly on the face and trunk. Some children are mildly listless and unwell, but others are quite happy to run around and play with others, despite quite a striking rash.

The important thing with chickenpox is to try to prevent the child from scratching the spots. The individual spots of chickenpox are fairly superficial and only involve the epidermis. This means that if they are left alone they will heal without scarring. If, however, the child scratches a chickenpox spot it is possible that scarring will result. It is therefore important to seek a doctor's advice about the best treatment for chickenpox spots. Very often a light calamine cream is all that is needed to control mild itch and prevent scratching.

SCARLET FEVER

The rash of scarlet fever is much finer than any of the others described above. The child usually has an all-over flushed appearance and is pinker than usual. The face is usually flushed, but there may be a rim of white skin around the mouth. The back of the mouth and the throat in the tonsil area is usually bright scarlet and the child is uncomfortable and complains of a sore throat. There is a high fever. As the rash fades, there is often striking peeling of the skin.

Children with scarlet fever should be encouraged to rest as much as possible, and the usual practice is to give them a 5-day course of an antibiotic syrup. This will help prevent the more serious complications of scarlet fever, including damage to the heart. If scarlet fever is suspected the family doctor should be called for a home visit without delay.

A number of other rarer childhood illnesses, usually due to viruses, are associated with a skin rash. In general the doctor should be consulted when children are fevered, listless, off their food, and always when they are in obvious pain.

CHILDHOOD INFECTIONS CONFINED TO THE SKIN

In addition to the generalized infectious diseases of childhood discussed above, childhood is a stage when a number of skin infections are more common than at other times in our lives. These skin infections include infection with the common wart virus, infection with bacteria causing impetigo, and other, rarer problems.

WARTS

Very few children manage to go through childhood without at some stage developing warts on the hands, face or feet. The Latin name for warts is *verruca*, and plantar warts, sometimes found on the soles of the feet, are often called verrucae. All warts are caused by an infective agent—a virus—but there are a number of different types of wart virus, which explains the very different appearances of warts on different parts of the skin.

The most common place for warts to develop is on the fingers around about the finger-nails. Many children have two or three small warts in this area. These warts frequently disappear of their own accord after 3–6 months and cause no problems. During this time the child may pass the wart virus to the hands of one of his or her friends or to a brother or sister, but as hand warts are so common it is almost impossible to prevent this happening.

No treatment for childhood warts can be carried out effectively without causing at least some discomfort, and at times quite a lot of pain. For this reason, and also because of the fact that in normal healthy children warts are usually self-limiting and will eventually clear of their own accord, many doctors are reluctant to embark on vigorous treatment. For many children the treatment of warts is their first encounter with a doctor or childrens' hospital. If the first contact is one that gives memories of pain, discomfort or being held firmly on mother's knee while an unpleasant burning material is applied to the warts, children will naturally develop a dislike and fear of both doctors and hospitals. For this reason, doctors are not enthusiastic about vigorous treatment of warts. Nevertheless, if a child has a large number of warts, if these warts are causing pain or discomfort, particularly around the nails, and if the warts have been present for 3–6 months and are showing no signs of disappearing, some treatment is probably justified and needed.

There are a number of wart paints on the market that contain materials designed to encourage peeling of the skin and minor irritation. These wart paints have been shown in scientific studies to be of some value. They are very safe and can be bought in the chemist's shop across the counter. It is worthwhile purchasing one of these wart paints and applying it regularly every night for a month or two to the warts before asking a doctor for more effective, but also more painful treatment.

Treatment for hand warts, if the wart paint preparations do not appear to be effective, consists of destroying the wart; this is usually done by freezing. Family doctors and specialists in hospitals use equipment designed to freeze the wart to very low temperatures. This can be temporarily extremely painful and uncomfortable, and it is no wonder that small children are frightened by the procedure. Freezing of warts is often done with liquid nitrogen, the temperature of which can be as low as $-70°C$. This may have to be applied to the wart not just once, but two or three times at intervals of 2–3 weeks. It is impossible to gauge with absolute accuracy the exact amount of freezing needed to destroy the wart but avoid damage to the surrounding skin. For this reason, many patients who have treatment with liquid nitrogen for warts will develop redness, and sometimes even blistering, of the surrounding skin a day or two after receiving liquid nitrogen treatment. If this should happen, the doctor who has given the treatment will give instructions as to what to do. It is best to prick the blister to remove the fluid, using a needle that has been sterilized in boiling water or in a flame, and then to cover the area with a clean, dry piece of elastoplast or other dressing. If blisters develop around a wart after freezing, do not assume that the doctor has done something wrong—people vary in the readiness with which blisters form, and this cannot be predicted in advance. The problem will settle down in a day or two. In the meantime, keep the area clean to avoid secondary infection.

Verrucae

Verrucae, or warts on the feet, tend to be more troublesome and frequently cause pain. They therefore require earlier and more vigorous treatment than hand warts (Figure 9). Many children develop verrucae, the wart virus often being picked up from the floor of the school gym or from the changing room at the local swimming pool. It is important to be fair to other parents and children, and to keep a child away from these public areas if he or she has plantar warts or verrucae. For children who are extremely sporty and keen to continue with their gymnastics, swimming, or other activities, plastic socks are available and can be used in these communal areas by individuals who have verrucae that are under treatment. The local swimming pool or sports centre may have specific regulations about the use of these plastic socks, so it is a good idea to make enquiries at an early stage.

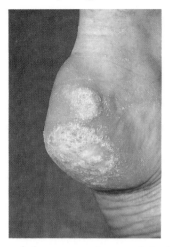

Figure 9 A cluster of plantar warts (veruccae) on the heel of a child.

Treatment for plantar warts is very similar to the treatment for hand warts. Because the thick skin of the sole of the foot tends to become heaped up over the top of the wart, it is often a good idea to use a sharp razor blade to very carefully remove just the top layer of the skin on the wart before applying a wart paint. Remember that this is to remove dead skin from the top of the wart, and not to cause bleeding. Applying a wart paint and a small plaster dressing on top may be effective, but if this does not clear the wart, once again, treatment by freezing may be carried out by the family doctor or local specialist. Very often, once one plantar wart develops, the child develops two or three more in the area of surrounding skin.

While the child is having treatment for plantar warts, spread of the wart virus to other family members should be avoided. The child should be prevented from running around the house with bare feet and encouraged to wear at least socks, and preferably slippers, to stop the wart virus being shed on the carpet of the bedroom or playroom for the next barefooted child along to pick up. Spread of the wart virus in the bathroom should also be avoided and the child with plantar warts should have his or her own towel and bath-mat. These suggestions may seem a nuisance, but if they prevent two or three other family members from developing painful warts, they are worthwhile.

Plane warts

Children occasionally develop small, rather flat warts on the face, particularly on the cheek. These are called plane warts and although they are much smaller than the warts found on the hands and on the feet, they are unusually difficult to treat and often sit stubbornly on the skin. Once again, the family doctor may not be enthusiastic about treating plane warts. The reason for this is that in time the child will develop immunity to the wart virus and the plane warts will disappear spontaneously, leaving no mark and no scarring. It is very difficult to treat plane warts without damaging the delicate facial skin and, particularly if freezing is carried out, scarring can result. It is therefore reasonable to delay treatment for warts for as long as possible, in the hope that nature will produce a perfect result without either pain or permanent scarring on the skin of the face.

Although it can be hard to accept when a child has large numbers of any type of wart, all warts on the skin of healthy people are self-limiting and will, in time, disappear without treatment when the affected person has developed immunity to the wart virus. The reasons for treating warts are that first this disappearance can take a long time, and secondly, that during this time the affected child may have considerable discomfort, particularly if the warts are around the finger-nails and on the sole of the foot. A third important reason is that warts are contagious, and one child can be responsible for a minor epidemic at home, in the school gym, or at the swimming pool.

IMPETIGO

Impetigo is a skin infection caused by bacteria. To many parents the word suggests that their child is in some way unclean or not well cared for. This is not the case, and it is important to realize that if any child has a cut or graze, particularly on the face, certain types of bacteria—mainly staphylococci and streptococci—can enter the abrasion and give rise to impetigo. This is usually recognized as a moist, weeping, crusted sore, often on the face around the mouth.

Impetigo responds very well to antibiotics, either applied as an ointment to the skin surface or as a syrup given by mouth for a few days. As it is particularly infectious it is important to ask the family doctor's advice if a child is suspected of having impetigo. Prompt treatment will result in complete cure, will prevent unsightly sores spreading over the child's skin, and will prevent transmission to other children.

An additional reason for asking for medical help without any delay is that a few children who develop impetigo also develop a kidney complaint as a result of the bacterial infection causing the impetigo. This reaction can cause serious kidney problems, but can be totally prevented if the child is given an appropriate antibiotic.

Although the rash of impetigo can be quite widespread, and can temporarily look very disfiguring, it affects only the most superficial layers of the epidermis. As this superficial epidermis is being renewed all the time (see Chapter 1), no permanent damage will be done to the child's skin—the impetigo lesions will heal with no scarring because the basal layer of keratinocytes is undamaged and will build a new and perfect epidermis. However, children should be prevented from scratching or picking at any lesions of impetigo, as this scratching or picking *can* damage the underlying dermis and could in turn give rise to scarring.

ECZEMA AND THE YOUNG SCHOOLCHILD

By far the most common type of childhood eczema is atopic eczema. Many babies with mild atopic eczema happily outgrow the problem before starting playgroup or school, but a few, often those with more severe eczema, still have problems. The young schoolchild with atopic eczema will have a dry skin and will often look a little pale and chronically tired, with small lines under the eyes. The parts of the body most involved are usually the face, hands around the wrists, the backs of the knees (Figure 10) and the elbows, but any part of the skin can be involved. Apart from using the treatments prescribed by the doctor or dermatologist, a lot can be done to help in practical everyday matters.

Cotton clothing is much the most comfortable for these children, and 100% cotton clothes can be bought from the large chain stores or from specialist shops. Children with atopic dermatitis benefit from as dust-free an environment as possible, and this can be created in the home, and particularly in the bedroom, by having

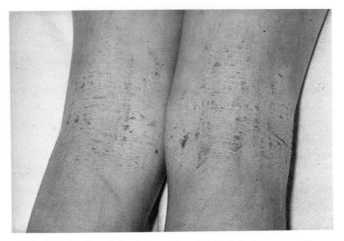

Figure 10　The backs of the knees of a child with severe atopic eczema, showing thickening of the skin and also scratch marks.

a wooden or linoleum-covered floor, not a fitted carpet, and a blind rather than curtains. The child's mattress should be in a plastic covering, as scales of skin work their way into a mattress and provide food for a very widespread problem—the house dust mite—which aggravates the skin of atopic dermatitis sufferers. The child's pillow and quilt should be of synthetic material rather than feather-filled, as many atopic children are irritated by feathers. Similarly, the hair of many animals will make the problem of atopic dermatitis more irritable, so a household with a bad atopic child should not have a hairy pet—much better not to start than to have the unhappy decision of deciding whether or not to give away a well-loved family friend. Play materials should neither wet the skin nor dry it out. Water play and the sandpit are two areas that should be avoided by the atopic child, as they will undoubtedly make the problem worse. Crayons and felt-tip pens are a better option.

Consider joining the National Eczema Society if you are a family with atopic eczema sufferers. The Society produces a large number of helpful leaflets dealing with practical problems of everyday life, and can offer an understanding, listening ear and support on the days a stressed mother with an unhappy, itchy child feels she just cannot cope with the situation.

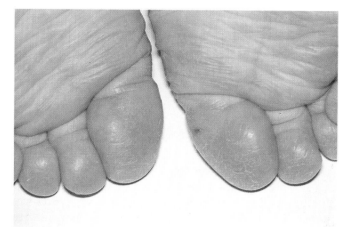

Figure 11 The shiny skin seen on the soles of the feet of a child with juvenile plantar dermatosis.

JUVENILE PLANTAR DERMATOSIS

Young children may develop shiny, scaly soles on their feet (see Figure 11), and may also develop painful hacks at this site. Some, but not all, of these children are also atopic, and most of them are active sporty children. The problem appears to be related to excess sweating, and can be helped by cotton socks, open sandals rather than trainers or wellington boots, and a cork insole in the shoe, although this may require shoes half a size larger than usual. The children usually outgrow this problem in 1–2 years.

4.

The teenager

The teenage years are often traumatic times. Major decisions have to be made about schools, future jobs, training courses, and University entrance. The teenager also has to come to terms with the changes in their body brought about by the hormonal changes of puberty, and learn to relate to other people of both sexes without the protective network of the family. All this has to be accomplished at a time when sudden unpredictable mood swings can make life difficult for everyone.

This is also a time of life when the skin is changing, sometimes quite dramatically, and the temporary presence of blemishes, perhaps not very obvious to anyone else, but that seem enormous to the teenager, can make an already traumatic situation even more difficult to bear.

NORMAL CHANGES IN THE SKIN'S BEHAVIOUR AT PUBERTY

The most obvious effects on the skin of the sudden surge of hormones through the bloodstream between the ages of about 10 and 14 are on the sebaceous, or grease-producing, glands and the hair. The sebaceous glands have lain dormant since birth but with the stimulus of hormones they suddenly become very active. These glands are found in their greatest numbers on the forehead, the nose, the central part of the cheeks, and the chin. This central panel of the face will become shiny and greasy because the sebum from these very active glands is coming to the skin surface through the small openings of the pilosebaceous follicles, see (p. 2) or 'pores'. If this sebum is regularly washed away with soap and water, the skin will usually remain smooth and healthy-looking, but in some teenagers the amount of sebum trying to get to the surface is so great that the opening of the follicle becomes blocked at the skin surface. This blockage quickly becomes blackened, as a result of exposure to the air, and the result is a blackhead. If this is not dealt with rapidly, it can be the beginning of acne. Girls will frequently find that their greasy skin is particularly troublesome in the week or so before their period is due.

The best specific aid to coping with teenage skin is regular use of soap and water. Teenage skin needs the drying effect of soap, and does not require greasy moisturizing agents or emollients.

There are many sebaceous glands in the scalp and as these are also activated by the circulating hormones, the hair will become greasy and lank if not shampooed frequently. Many teenagers wish to shampoo their hair daily, and this will do no harm. There are a number of shampoos available for frequent or daily use. These contain less drying detergent than other brands, and are recommended. No shampoo will ever stop the activity of the sebaceous glands, but a beneficial effect of this activity is that teenage hair, if kept clean, is usually beautifully glossy without the addition of expensive cream rinses or conditioners.

Teenage skin miseries can be partly controlled, if not completely prevented, by a sensible lifestyle. Although this is much easier said than done, a balanced diet, regular mealtimes, plenty of fresh fruit and vegetables, half-an-hour in the fresh air each day and a regular exercise programme are all good for the body in general, including the skin. Late nights, stuffy discos and a diet of sweets and chips do not help anyone to look their best.

The combination of hormone activity and new, stressful situations will also stimulate the apocrine glands in the armpits to become active. In childhood these glands are not active, but now a deodorant or antiperspirant will be needed. Do not imagine that these preparations do any harm by blocking the activity of the apocrine glands. The glands are very small, and no harm whatever is done by stopping their activity.

COSMETICS AND MAKE-UP FOR TEENAGE SKIN

This is a time of life for experimenting, and investigating the ranges of make-up and cosmetics available is part of the fun. In general, modern cosmetics do no harm, and many do the skin a lot of good, in addition to being decorative. However, it is worth remembering that, in general, the best approach to make-up is to use it to help what already looks good to look even better, rather than to use it as a mask to cover up underlying spots and blackheads. Skin preparations for teenage or oily skin should be used, not the heavy, greasy preparations aimed at older people whose skins may require extra grease.

Some make-up aimed at young skin is oil-free and based on a water and powder mixture. This washes off easily, so special cleansers are unlikely to be needed. Some of the special cover sticks are very effective for individual temporary spots and, because they contain drying agents and antiseptics, will also speed up the disappearance of individual spots. However, these should not be used daily or on several spots. If this situation develops, a more specific treatment for acne, discussed below, is required. If heavier make-up is used, it is important to have a regular routine for its removal at the end of the day. Otherwise the skin will become clogged, sallow, and spots are likely.

Most facial make-up needs to be removed with a cleansing lotion, as ordinary soap will not do a proper job. A cleanser that makes the skin feel clean and soft, but not greasy, should be used every night. If the skin is particularly greasy and an evening out is planned, it may be necessary to use this cleanser in the early evening and apply fresh make-up. Piling a new layer of make-up on top of an old one is not a good idea—the skin will look caked and spots will be encouraged. When eye make-up is used, a special eye make-up remover will be needed.

More exotic experiments may involve the use of fluorescent face paints, some of which contain a sun-screen. These seem to be particularly popular on ski slopes, and can look very dramatic. Remember that the skin not covered with face paint also needs some protection, or the face will be covered in sunburned stripes the next day.

SKIN PROBLEMS COMMON IN TEENAGERS

The particular skin problems of teenagers are usually acne and problems associated with sporting activities, for example athlete's foot (see p. 51). The teenage years are the time of life when most

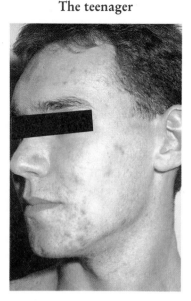

Figure 12 Mild facial acne.

moles appear and, for an unlucky few, the problems of eczema are still around.

ACNE

Studies on teenagers in the UK have suggested that it is normal rather than abnormal to have at least a mild degree of acne, which is not usually called acne at all but just thought of as a few spots at some time during the teenage years. The problem usually begins earlier with girls than with boys. Girls will find their acne problems more troublesome between the ages of 13 and 16, while for many boys the problem does not start until about 15 and goes on until the age of about 19. Some people suffer from lingering problems with acne after the teenage years, but this is the exception rather than the rule.

Mild acne usually involves the face, and the area most commonly affected is the central panel—the forehead, the nose, and the chin (Figure 12). Many teenagers have a few blackheads in these areas. As described earlier (see p. 42), blackheads are the result of the obstruction of the outflow of sebum from hair follicles opening onto the face. If the problem with obstructed outflow continues, the sebum trapped on the way to the surface of the epidermis may leak into the surrounding dermis. When this happens the problem changes from being just a simple blackhead to being a raised, inflamed papule or spot on the skin. Sometimes these red spots develop unsightly yellow heads. As well as involving the face, acne may involve the front of the chest and, particularly in boys, the back over the shoulder area.

Nowadays, almost all grades of acne can be controlled, if not prevented. Mild acne can usually be managed quite well by the teenager, with the help of advice from the local chemist. More stubborn, extensive or persistent acne will probably need the help of the family doctor, and a few patients with acne will require referral to a specialist dermatologist. Nevertheless, no-one should consider that acne is a minor problem, either to be ignored or to be the subject of unkind jokes. To the teenager it is a major problem and treating the acne when it is not too obvious will prevent the problem progressing to severe acne, which requires more intensive treatment. In the past it was not always possible to improve every severity of acne, and even now some adults have scars on their faces and backs as the result of acne activity when teenagers. Advances in our understanding and management of acne in the past 10 years mean that this should no longer occur.

Mild acne

Mild acne will affect any teenager who has a particularly greasy skin. If the skin is always shiny and greasy-looking, and if the hair is also very greasy, regular washing will do a lot to prevent acne developing. This means washing two or three times a day with soap and warm water, thorough rinsing with fresh water, and gently patting dry with a towel. As stated earlier, hair can be very greasy at this stage in life, and hair styles should be chosen so that they are off the face and do not lie on the forehead, which can create a very greasy environment on which blackheads will develop.

If, despite regular washing, a few acne spots develop, the local chemist will be able to advise on appropriate mild acne treatments designed to dry the skin, and often containing an antiseptic to prevent any secondary infection.

Try not to pick, squeeze or otherwise fiddle with either black-heads or acne spots. This almost always makes the situation look worse and, although it can be difficult advice to follow, finger-nails should never be used. Blackhead extractors are sold by the major chemists but must be used with care and should always be sterilized in boiling water after use. They should not be used just before going out to meet friends, as for an hour or two after applying pressure to the skin around blackheads and spots, the skin will be inflamed and red.

Treatment

If acne persists and becomes more widespread, the family doctor should be asked for help. Treatment for acne can involve preparations applied directly to the skin and oral tablets.

Benzoyl peroxide Treatments applied to the skin are very often based on **benzoyl peroxide**, which is a drying, mildly antiseptic preparation. Very often, when this is first used it can cause some dryness, redness and minor irritation. This is part of the treatment, and the preparation should not be stopped because this happens. After about a week the redness usually disappears, as do the blackheads.

Antibiotics Another approach to managing mild acne is the use of oral antibiotics. These are prescribed not because acne is an infection, but because of their other benefits—among other things, antibiotics appear to alter the movement of the white cells normally found in the blood vessels. It is these white cells—**leucocytes**—that are responsible for the yellow tops of spots on the skin. By altering the way in which they move into the skin, antibiotics make inflamed spots less likely.

The doctor will usually prescribe a tetracycline antibiotic for the treatment of acne. However, tetracycline should not be prescribed if there is any possibility of pregnancy, because it can cause a yellow stain on both the bones and the teeth of the unborn baby; alternative antibiotics can be prescribed if pregnancy is a possibility.

As with all medicines, it is essential to take tetracycline in the way in which it will be most effective. Ideally, it should be taken with a glass of water half-an-hour or so before a meal, so that it can be absorbed through the lining of the stomach; if it is taken with food it may not be absorbed and may therefore not be of any value. One of the most common reasons for patients with acne being disappointed with their antibiotic is because they are not taking the antibiotic in the manner prescribed.

Acne does not respond immediately to treatment. Treatment applied directly to the skin usually takes a week or two to have an effect, and the usual waiting time for an oral antibiotic is 1–2 months. The way in which antibiotics are prescribed for acne is quite different to the way in which they are prescribed for true infectious diseases. In infectious diseases, a high dose of the antibiotic is prescribed for a short period of time. In contrast, for acne, a relatively low dose of antibiotic is prescribed for a long period of time. Many acne sufferers have to take tetracyclines for 6, 9 or even 12 months. Fortunately, tetracyclines are safe preparations and there are no long-term side-effects. An additional advantage of tetracycline is that it is now rarely used for problems other than acne. There is therefore no risk that its long-term use for acne will result in bacteria or other organisms becoming resistant to its action, causing problems if an antibiotic is needed later in life.

An alternative way of using antibiotics is to apply them directly to the skin surface; this can be done with tetracycline and erythromycin. These topical antibiotics are of some benefit to acne sufferers, but are not usually as effective as when the antibiotic is taken by mouth.

Specialist treatment　If acne does not respond to a variety of prescribed topical preparations applied to the skin in combination with antibiotics, the family doctor may well refer the patient to a specialist dermatologist for advice. There are two main additional approaches to the treatment of acne over and above those already mentioned.

For girls there is the possibility of hormonal adjustment. Many girls find that their acne flares in the week before their period because the sebaceous glands are stimulated by circulating hormones (see p. 42). For this reason, the use of a hormonal combination similar to that found in the oral contraceptive pill may well be of value in the management of acne. The hormonal combination most commonly prescribed for acne is Dianette, and it is taken in a way similar to the oral contraceptive, starting 5 days after the period has begun and continuing for 21–22 days. As with other forms of treatment for acne, there is usually a lag period of 2 to 3 months before any benefit can be expected. Most doctors who prescribe hormonal treatment for acne prefer girls to discontinue it after 9 months to a year, to be sure that their own hormones are still working in the normal manner. It is also important to have an occasional examination of the breast tissue when taking hormonal treatment in this way, as small cysts are more common in those who are receiving hormonal therapy. With these two precautions, Dianette can be very helpful for the girl with persistent acne.

An alternative treatment for acne in both sexes is a synthetic, vitamin A-like drug called Roaccutane in Europe and Acutane in the US. This has a very dramatic effect on the sebaceous glands. If small samples of skin are removed before and 4 months after oral Roaccutane and compared under a microscope, it will be seen that after Roaccutane treatment the sebaceous glands have shrunk dramatically to a size similar to that found in small children before puberty. As the sebaceous glands shrink, their secretion of sebum dries up. Thus, the effect of Roaccutane is to cause a dramatic shutdown of the activity of the sebaceous gland responsible for acne, which results in a drying of the skin surface.

In addition, however, Roaccutane also has an effect on all the other grease-producing and lubricating glands of the body. The lips tend to dry and crack in the way which they may do when exposed to cold winter weather, and the lining of the nose may become dry, giving a permanent feeling of a stuffy nose and sometimes resulting in nose bleeds. The secretion of tears is also affected and there are complaints of dry-feeling, gritty eyes.

A further, but also temporary, problem that may develop while on Roaccutane treatment is that the level of circulating fats in the blood may become elevated. It is rare to have to cut treatment short because of this, and the levels return rapidly to their pretreatment state, but it is necessary to have a blood sample checked, usually on an empty stomach.

All of these side-effects of Roaccutane are relatively easy to put up with provided the acne sufferer has severe acne and knows that the treatment is doing good. Very much more serious, however, is the fact that Roaccutane can damage an unborn child if taken by a young woman who is in the early stages of pregnancy, resulting in very serious defects of the heart, the hearing system and other organs. For this reason, it is *absolutely essential* that Roaccutane is not given to any young girl in whom there is even the most remote possibility of a pregnancy, either already started at the time Roaccutane is prescribed for her or if there is a possibility that she might become pregnant while on the course of Roaccutane, or for a month or so after stopping treatment.

A standard course of Roaccutane usually lasts 4 months and the risk to an unborn child is so serious that most specialists will not prescribe Roaccutane unless the girl who wishes treatment for her acne is prepared to take the oral contraceptive for a month before starting Roaccutane, continue the oral contraceptive for the full 4 months of Roaccutane treatment and for another month after the Roaccutane course ends. Thus a 4-month course of Roaccutane involves a 6-month course of treatment with an oral contraceptive.

Roaccutane is a very effective method of treating severe acne but because of the serious potential problem of damage to an unborn child, it is not a drug that is prescribed lightly. In the UK it can be prescribed only by specialists through a hospital pharmacy, and the family doctor will therefore need to refer the patient for a specialist opinion if they feel that acne is severe enough to merit Roaccutane treatment.

Once Roaccutane treatment is discontinued, most acne sufferers find that their acne has greatly improved and that this improvement is maintained for a year or more after completion of the 4-month course. Occasionally a second course is needed but, provided that the same precautions are taken as before, this can be prescribed.

In summary, teenage acne vulgaris is very common in a minor form. Sensible skin care and prompt attention to mild acne should prevent the problem progressing to a more severe form. There is a little evidence to suggest that severe acne runs in families, and therefore if either parent or an older brother or sister had severe acne, it is a good idea for the young teenager to be particularly careful about the care of his or her skin, and to try to prevent the same problem developing.

SPORT

A large number of dermatological problems may arise in association with sporting activities. Regular exercise of some type is known to help general health and appearance of the skin at any age. The teenage years are a good time to try out various types of sport, and to decide which ones will become a lifetime habit. Because the use of swimming pools, changing facilities, and gymnasium floors, which are shared by many people who prefer to do their aerobics or yoga barefoot can lead to spread of infection, it is important to be particularly careful about personal cleanliness and thus prevent the spreading of infection to others.

The most common problems associated with sporting activity are fungal infections, and the most common of these is **athlete's foot**, which develops between the toe webs and may also involve the nails.

ATHLETE'S FOOT

This problem is caused by small fungi that live on tiny scraps of skin. As the skin is constantly being shed, small particles of skin may be rubbed from the soles of the feet onto the floors of changing rooms, swimming pools, etc. and may then be picked up by the next person who walks over the area. Fungi may live in these scraps of skin and can give rise to problems. The first sign that an individual has athlete's foot is usually the presence of white, blotting paper-like skin in the toe webs, most commonly in the web between the fourth and fifth toe. This may become very itchy and sometimes there is an associated unpleasant smell. Scratching will cause inflammation and bleeding. The infection will sometimes involve the instep area rather more than the toe webs, but this is not so frequent.

If the skin infection is recognized and treated promptly, it can usually be cleared relatively easily. If, however, the infection on the skin is not recognized or is ignored, the same fungal infection may spread to involve the nails. When this happens the nail becomes rough, crumbles, and develops irregular white patches. As time goes by the nail may become very thick and difficult to cut. This can lead to pain and difficulty finding comfortable shoes.

Once the nails are involved with fungal infection, curing the problem is very much more difficult. It takes from 1 to 2 years for a toe-nail to grow right out, and treatment for fungal infection of the toe-nail needs to be continued for this entire period of time. Even then it is very easy to re-infect toe-nails from shoes, and many people who developed fungal infection of toe-nails when they were teenagers still have the problem 20, 30 and even 40 years later. It is therefore important to be aware of the possible problem of athlete's foot, to know what to look for, and to take prompt action if the skin appears to be involved. If this is done it is unlikely that fungal infection of the toe-nails will develop.

OTHER FUNGAL INFECTIONS

Fungal infection does not involve only the feet, although this is by far the most common site. Individuals who are exposed to cattle with a fungal infection called cattle ringworm (a circular patch on the skin due to a fungal infection and not, as the name might suggest, to a worm) may develop a rather more acute fungal infection on any part of the skin that has been in contact with cattle. In children this may involve the scalp and can give rise to a rather dramatic, oozing, infected-looking area. In addition, the fungus that causes athlete's foot can occasionally cause problems elsewhere on the body, leaving circular, slightly red, scaling areas. This is called **tinea corporis**, and may be due to infection either spread from one human to another or spread from the family pet.

PREVENTION AND TREATMENT OF FUNGAL INFECTION

Good hygiene should prevent the great majority of fungal infections of the skin from ever developing. After using communal bathing, showering and changing facilities, the skin should be dried thoroughly, including the toe web area, and it is a good idea to use an antifungal dusting powder both on the feet and dusted into the socks and training shoes.

If white, peeling skin between the toes does occur, antifungal dusting powders and creams can be bought over the counter from the chemist and will usually clear the problem. If, however, the problem persists after a week or two of such treatment, and particularly if the area involved is itchy and red, the family doctor should be consulted. It may be necessary to take a small scraping of skin and send it to the laboratory to confirm the fungal infection. This involves removing the dead surface of skin with a blade. It is not painful and can be compared to cutting the hair or nails.

If the family doctor is fairly certain that there is a fungal infection, they may prescribe one of the very effective modern antifungal creams or ointments. If this is *not* effective, and particularly if the infection is on a part of the body other than between the toes, the doctor may prescribe a course of oral antifungal tablets. This will not usually be done until after an adequate trial of treatment with creams or ointments.

For many years the most effective oral treatment available was **griseofulvin**. This was very effective in the treatment of infections of the skin, although less effective for treatment of the nails. At the present time there are some exciting new developments in the treatment of fungal infection of the skin, and newer drugs which are very effective in the treatment of fungal infection of the nail, are now becoming available. One of these is **terbinafine** (Lamisil).

BLISTERS

Other skin problems associated with sporting activities include friction and chafing, sometimes even blisters, caused by ill-fitting footwear. Sports shoes should be comfortable for the sport being played. Trainers have recently become a high-fashion item rather than the practical sporty shoes that they were originally intended to be and although a particular brand and colour may be good for the image, they may not be the size and type of shoe correct for the particular sport. Enthusiastic half marathon runners will need a much higher quality shoe than the occasional tennis player. Take the advice of a good sports store, and do not insist on the brand that everyone else is wearing if it is not the type of shoe that is best for you.

THE COLD SORE VIRUS

Enthusiastic rugby players and others who play contact sports may occasionally develop problems with the herpes simplex or **cold sore virus**, which is passed direct from skin to skin in, for example, the rugby scrum. The rather unattractive name for this is, perhaps not surprisingly, scrum pox. Cold sore sufferers, should try to prevent skin-to-skin contact until the cold sore has healed.

MOLES (MELANOCYTIC NAEVI)

Between the ages of 12 and 20 it is normal to develop a sprinkling of small, flat, brown marks on the skin surface. Most of these are

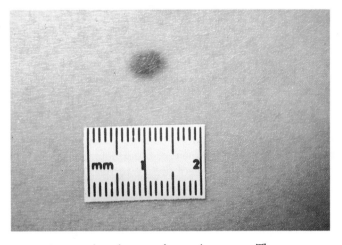

Figure 13   A normal mole or melanocytic naevus. The average young adult has 20–40 of these.

found on skin surfaces that are exposed to sunlight, and will be seen mainly on the upper arms in both sexes, on the legs in girls and on the back in boys. These small moles are entirely normal. The great majority are smaller than 3–4 mm in diameter and can easily be covered by the blunt end of a pencil (Figure 13). The average young adult in North America and the UK has between 20 and 40 of these small moles scattered over his or her skin. They are entirely normal and the vast majority will remain present on the skin for around 20 years and will then slowly disappear in middle age. Older people have very few moles on their skin.

Some people are confused about what is a mole and what is a freckle. This can be difficult but, in general, freckles are found mostly on the face, and become much more obvious in the summer. In the winter they may disappear completely. Small children often have lots of freckles on their faces, but very few moles elsewhere. Moles do not disappear completely in the winter, although they may become much less obvious.

Occasionally, particularly in boys, an interesting halo of white skin appears round a small mole. This most often happens on the back, and is usually seen or recognized in the summer months when the surrounding skin has a sun-tan and the mole is sitting in a little circle of white skin. This is called a **halo naevus** (Figure 14) and, once again,

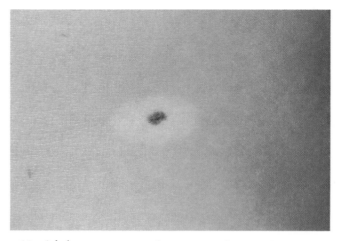

Figure 14 A halo naevus at an early stage. In a few months this mole will disappear, leaving a pale area on the skin. It will take months or even years for the natural colour to return.

is nothing to worry about. For reasons we do not understand, this particular naevus or mole has been recognized by the body as being different from the rest of the body, and the body's immune defences have mounted an attack on the pigment-producing cells that make up the mole. These have developed from the melanocytes—the pigment-producing cells found in the lower layer of the epidermis. If the halo naevus is observed for a few months, the central mole will be seen to change from brown to pink, and then to disappear completely. The white area that is left when the mole disappears will persist for some time, often 2 or 3 years, before the normal skin colour returns. During this time, it is particularly important to protect this area from strong sun-light, as all the pigment-producing melanocytes in the area have temporarily disappeared and the skin may become quite badly burned if it is not adequately protected.

Occasionally, moles become inflamed and lumpy. This most often happens to moles on the face, particularly if the mole has one or two protruding hairs. The reason for this sudden inflammation is often that the hair follicle has become irritated and inflamed. If this happens regularly, the doctor may decide that it is best to remove the mole. This involves a small operation under a local anaesthetic, and may leave a small scar.

TEENAGE ECZEMA

Most children who have atopic eczema as babies grow out of it before they are aged 5 but an unlucky few still have teenage problems, although there is still every reason to hope that they also will eventually grow out of it. In the meantime the skin should be treated gently. Unlike most teenagers, the skin will probably be dry rather than oily. One of the compensations of having teenage eczema is that acne will almost certainly not occur. The skin should be prevented from drying out by having a warm—not hot—daily bath with an added emollient. Baths are better for dry skin than showers, as there is more time for the emollients to work on the skin. A cleansing ointment (such as emulsifying ointment BP or Unguentum Merck) should be used instead of soap and creams may be prescribed by the family doctor or specialist. Many teenagers get very tired of daily skin care for their eczema and some just give up in despair; this should be avoided.

5.

The young adult

Once the turbulent teenage years are over, the skin usually settles down and is really very little problem for most people for the next decade or two. Three areas that can give rise to problems in the twenties and thirties are minor changes in the skin's activity during pregnancy, which are noticed by some women, and, for both sexes, possible problems with dermatitis arising as a result of exposure to substances either at home or in the course of their occupation. In addition, psoriasis often presents for the first time in this age group.

SKIN CHANGES ASSOCIATED WITH PREGNANCY

During pregnancy, the levels of circulating female hormones in the body are very much higher than normal. The skin is responsive to these hormones and, in general, the skin changes of pregnancy are flattering—most women feel that their skin is fresher and smoother-looking than before, and are very happy with the effect of their circulating hormones. Occasionally, in the first 3 months of pregnancy some women experience a temporary flare-up of acne, particularly if this has affected them earlier in life. This is usually a passing phase and will disappear at about the same time as morning sickness.

A high proportion of the hair on the scalp is in the active growing phase during pregnancy, and for this reason hair during pregnancy is often particularly thick, lustrous and healthy-looking. This is a pleasant bonus for the pregnant woman, but unfortunately she will pay for it after the baby is born, as about 3 months after the birth much of the hair that was growing during pregnancy will switch into its normal shedding phase. The mother may be alarmed to see an unexpectedly high number of hairs in the basin or shower when washing her hair and, if she tugs gently at her scalp hair, she will find that quite a few hairs are easily pulled away. This is an entirely normal effect of the hormonal changes in the woman's body after delivery and there is no way of preventing it. After the active growing phase, the hair follicles naturally progress to the resting phase, resulting in shedding of scalp hair. For a few months the scalp hair will be a little thinner than normal, but in time the normal rhythm of hair growth and shedding will return. Although the woman herself may be acutely aware of her thinner hair it is not usually noticeable to anyone else. Over this period she should wash her hair gently with a mild shampoo and should not use harsh brushes and combs. The hair may look thicker if a short hair-style is adopted. A new perm is best delayed until the hair starts to thicken up again.

The pigment-producing melanocytes of the skin are also mildly sensitive to female hormones. In most women this does not produce a visible change in the pigmentation of the body, but in women with darker, hispanic or Mediterranean-type colouring, there are often quite striking changes in the skin's pigmentation during pregnancy. There is pigmentation on the mid-line of the skin of the stomach, around the nipples, and possibly around the cheeks and mouth. The medical term for this facial pigmentation is '**chloasma**' or, more descriptively, 'the mask of pregnancy'. It is often made more striking by exposure to the sun, as the effects of circulating hormones add to the effect of the sun and stimulate the pigment-producing properties of the melanocytes. This pigmentation will fade after delivery of the baby but does not always disappear completely. If problems with facial pigmentation were experienced in one pregnancy, it is a good idea to try to avoid excessive sun exposure and to use a sun-block when expecting the next baby, although even this may not completely prevent the development of some degree of pigmentation.

During pregnancy, many women find that their skin becomes slightly drier than usual. This will pass after delivery of the baby, but in the meantime a pleasant bath oil and possibly one of the cleansing ointments, such as emulsifying ointment BP, instead of soap for the body and a cosmetic cleansing preparation for the face can be used.

DERMATITIS

There are many different kinds of dermatitis. We have already discussed the common problem of atopic eczema or atopic derma-

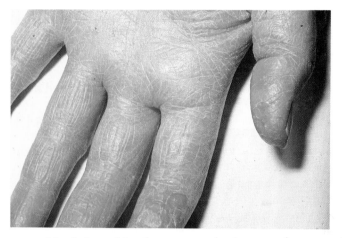

Figure 15 Hand dermatitis of a person who is exposed to excessive detergents and water.

titis (see p. 25), which is most common in young children and becomes steadily less common in older people.

Contact dermatitis is also very common and may be due either to a substance or conditions that irritates everyone's skin—**irritant dermatitis**—or to a specific personal allergy to the specific material that is causing the problem—**allergic contact dermatitis.**

IRRITANT DERMATITIS

This is particularly common in young mothers and in others whose work or hobbies involve them in exposing their hands to water and degreasing agents such as detergents. People who have to do a great deal of dish- or clothes-washing by hand and who use strong detergents and possibly also special nappy-cleaning agents, may find that their hands are red, dry, and chapped (Figure 15). This may be particularly marked under rings. It is not because of an allergy to the metal of which the rings are made, but because some detergent material may lodge there and not be rinsed away, even by a brisk rinsing of the hands under the tap after carrying out the washing.

Other people who are likely to get irritant dermatitis are those whose jobs involve contact with oil, for example garage mechanics.

Here the problem is usually the fact that strong degreasing agents have to be used to clean hands after the day's work. Special cleaners are often used. These work very well but remove the protective layer of oil and lipid from the skin surface. In time, therefore, the hands become dry, easily cracked and, in cold weather, the skin surface may break down, with uncomfortable cracks and fissures.

Irritant dermatitis can be prevented by commonsense measures. Remember that skin can only put up with so much. If your occupation, hobby, or domestic life involves a lot of washing or exposing your hands to soap, detergents and water, make it a lifetime habit to use waterproof gloves for wet work. Both rubber and vinyl gloves are readily available. Vinyl gloves are preferable, as some people may develop a contact sensitivity to rubber, whereas allergic reactions to vinyl are rare. Those who have never used gloves when their hands are in water may feel at first that they will be a nuisance and will make them clumsy. However, after a few days of regular use it is easy to adjust to using them.

The best way to use vinyl gloves is to wear a thin pair of cotton gloves, sometimes called household gloves (available in larger chemists and drug stores) under a relatively inexpensive pair of unlined vinyl gloves. Some people prefer to use flock-lined vinyl gloves, but it is very easy for some hot soapy water to trickle down inside these gloves and, once the lining has become damp and sodden with detergent, they can be very uncomfortable to wear. If a combination of a vinyl outer glove and a thin cotton inner glove is used the cotton gloves can be rinsed out and dried after use if the inside of the gloves has become damp and contaminated with detergent.

Exposure of the skin of the hands to hot water and detergents is also, of course, reduced by automatic washing machines and dishwashers, but even with these it is difficult to avoid completely the drying effects of soap and water particularly in some occupations, such as nursing, or if there is a young family.

An important habit to adopt is the regular use of a good hand cream. Throughout adult life the grease-producing glands of the skin slowly become less active, until in old age, grease and lipid must be constantly replaced on the body's entire skin surface because the grease-producing glands can no longer do this work themselves (see p. 70). The skin on the hands, particularly the backs of the hands, does not have a rich supply of sebaceous glands and this is the area of our body that is most constantly subjected to the degreasing effect of harsh weather, detergents and other trauma. People who have an occupation involving a lot of washing, or an outdoor hobby such as car maintenance, gardening or fishing, often develop very uncomfortable dry hands with hacks on the fingertips. Regular use of hand cream will cure this problem and prevent it developing again. A hand cream should be easy to use and should be applied at the end of each day. If dry, sore hands are particularly troublesome, a small tube of hand cream can be kept in the pocket and applied regularly throughout the day after washing the hands. This routine will very quickly restore the hands to normal, and will make dry, red, wrinkled hands feel more comfortable and also look much more attractive. Many ranges of hand cream are now available and are aimed at both sexes.

ALLERGIC CONTACT DERMATITIS

This type of contact dermatitis often first appears in the twenties. It is much less common than irritant dermatitis, but it is also a considerable inconvenience. In allergic contact dermatitis, for reasons that we do not yet completely understand, the body develops a specific immunological or allergic reaction against a substance that most people can handle with no problem. A good example of such a substance is nickel, which is found in many of the materials handled all the time in the course of the working day. Cutlery contains nickel, even if it is labelled stainless steel, and it is in coins, spectacle frames, bicycle handlebars, front door keys, and most jewellery. Most of us handle all these things with no problem, but around 10% of the population develop a sore, itchy rash when they handle nickel.

One difficulty about identifying the cause of an allergic contact dermatitis is the fact that the areas that develop the rash are not always those that are most commonly in contact with the material causing it. Thus, although the hands and the area under a metal wrist-watch are often involved in nickel dermatitis, there may also be unexpected and initially puzzling involvement of, for example, the eyelids.

If sore, red, itchy areas develop on the skin of any part of the body, and if these do not respond to commonsense treatment with gentle cleansing and the use of a good hand cream or

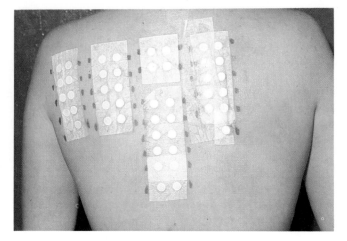

Figure 16 The appearance of the back while carrying out patch testing for contact dermatitis.

moisturizing cream, a doctor should be consulted. They may be able to identify the likely problem and, if they think that an allergic contact dermatitis is possible, they may carry out some special patch tests on your back, or make a referral to a specialist to have this done.

Patch testing

Patch tests involve putting a very small quantity of the material or materials most likely to cause allergic dermatitis on the back, in a specially designed type of dressing (see Figure 16). This is removed after 48 hours, the area is examined, and is then inspected again 48 hours later. Therefore on the week patch testing is carried out you need to be available to see the doctor for a short time on three alternate days. A small, red, mildly itchy area will identify the areas of skin that have been in contact with a material to which there is a specific allergy.

This technique at first seems suitable for self-administration at home, but in practice the results are difficult to interpret. The diagnosis of allergic contact dermatitis should be made by specialists.

If an allergic contact dermatitis to, for example, nickel is found the doctor or specialist will produce a long list of materials that should be avoided. This will be very much easier said than done,

Table 2 Common causes of allergic contact dermatitis (not a complete list)

Material causing dermatitis	Most common site problem
Nickel	Hands and areas in contact with nickel, e.g. under watch-strap and ear-rings
Material used in curing or colouring leather	Feet—from shoes
Rubber and related chemicals	Anywhere, commonly the face
Plants, e.g. *Primula obconica*	Face from airborne material Hands from contact
Fragrances	Face from cosmetics Entire body from washing powders
Preservative used in creams and ointments	Areas of skin to which creams are applied, especially around leg ulcers

but many helpful hints are available such as coating keys and cutlery handles with plastic.

Sometimes, when an allergy like this has first been diagnosed and a two-page list of all the common materials not to touch has been produced, it is easy to despair and to decide that it is too difficult to carry out the advice offered and that you will not even attempt to do so, but will just live with the problem. This is not advisable. Even avoiding the materials that cause problems *most* of the time will help the skin. If the advice is too difficult, or even impossible, the doctor should be consulted. In the UK, specially trained nurses and health visitors can offer practical advice and support for dealing with this kind of problem. People on a low income may be able to obtain financial support to replace items of furniture, for example.

Other fairly common causes of dermatitis are shown in Table 2. Materials used to make shoes quite often cause problems, which can be due to the dye used in colouring the shoes, to the material used in curing the leather, or to the glues used to fit the various pieces of a shoe together. Once it is established exactly which component of the shoes is causing the problem, practical advice on suitable brands of shoes and alternative materials in shoes that will not cause you problems can be given. Most shoe manufacturers are very helpful in giving full information on the constituents used in each model of shoe and the local dermatologist who specializes in contact dermatitis may have this list already available.

Another interesting and fairly common cause of dermatitis is the household plant *Primula obconica*. These quite popular plants can be bought in most garden centres and many supermarkets. They can cause a very acute and severe redness and puffiness of the face, hands and other exposed areas as the result of fine hairs, which become detached from the leaves of the plant and float off into the air around it. Most people who develop a primula dermatitis think at first that the problem is due to something they have put on their face, such as make-up, because they are not aware of these tiny particles circulating in the air.

Other materials that are fairly common causes of problems include chrome, used in the building industry, which can be a problem for many men working in labouring jobs, and perfumes. Perfumes are not just found in expensive little bottles; fragrances are used in a great many everyday materials, such as soap, shampoo, washing powder, fabric conditioner, and cosmetics. If a sensitivity to perfumes develops, fragrance-free, low allergen or low allergy materials are a great help.

Sometimes allergic contact dermatitis is caused by handling material in the course of one's daily work. In this case the factory medical officer or a similar person may be involved and can be extremely helpful. These people are used to dealing with this kind of problem, and it is often possible for the affected individual to be moved around the work area so that they can continue to be employed by the same company but need no longer handle the material that caused the problems. Other helpful individuals are the family doctor and the industrial medical liaison officer. Help from these people is more constructive than a decision to leave the employment in which the dermatitis problem developed.

PSORIASIS

One of the most common problems seen by specialists is a scaly skin disease called **psoriasis**. This disease affects as many as one

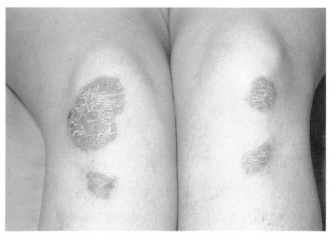

Figure 17 Typical lesions of psoriasis on the knees.

person in fifty in North America and Europe. The UK television programme *The Singing Detective* had as the central character a man with a very severe psoriasis, and this did much to raise the awareness of the disease in the general population. However, the severity of the psoriasis experienced by this character led many people to believe that psoriasis is always a serious and crippling problem. In fact, most people who have psoriasis have a relatively mild problem. There is usually some scaling of the scalp, rather like severe dandruff, and some mild redness and scaling of the skin over the elbows, the knees, and sometimes the lower back (Figure 17). It affects both men and women, and there is usually a family tendency. Psoriasis is *not* an infectious problem, it cannot be transmitted by skin contact. It is not a form of skin cancer and neither does having psoriasis make it more likely that skin cancer will develop in the future.

A small number of drugs and medicines taken for quite separate problems may make psoriasis worse, and can also cause it for the first time. These include some antimalarial tablets needed when on holiday or living in tropical countries, and some medication used for the treatment of high blood pressure.

In addition to drugs and medicines, psoriasis is one of the conditions that is believed to be made worse, or that is actually brought on for the first time, by stress. A great many skin diseases are thought to be aggravated by stress but as it is very difficult to measure stress levels it is thus difficult to prove or disprove this theory and certain situations that are acutely stressful in one individual are regarded as relatively normal by another. However, the frequency with which psoriasis either appears for the first time or gets worse after important life events such as examinations, problems with employment, domestic and social problems, and bereavement all contribute to the current belief that stress does add to the problems of psoriasis sufferers.

Managing psoriasis

Mild psoriasis is often managed quite easily without medical supervision. A shampoo designed to remove scale from the scalp, for example Polytar or Capasal, and a simple ointment, for example white soft paraffin, after a bath or shower, will remove the excessive scaling. If this is not effective, family doctors and specialists have a wide range of ointments available. In the past decade the range of treatments available for people with psoriasis has expanded tremendously. These can be either creams or ointments, which are the usual basic treatment for most patients with psoriasis, or, for more severe cases, the use of tablets or injections.

Some older people reading this book who have had psoriasis for many years may have given up any kind of treatment because when they last asked for help they found the treatments available difficult to use, messy, or ineffective. If you have psoriasis and have not asked your doctor about treatment for 5 years or more, do go back discuss the newer treatments available. Advances in treatment in the past 10 years have made cleaner, safer, more effective creams and ointments available.

At present, we can control, but not cure, psoriasis. Regular treatment to the skin morning or evening will frequently be needed and, if used as suggested, will in most cases keep psoriasis almost invisible and make the skin feel much more comfortable. Psoriasis is not usually a painful disease, but the skin usually feels slightly tight, rather sensitive, and sometimes mildly itchy.

Most psoriasis sufferers find that their skin improves a lot when they are exposed to natural sunlight, for example when on holiday. Because of this beneficial effect, the family doctor may arrange a 6-week course of artificial sunlight during the winter months. However, when on holiday sun-bathing should not be overdone to the extent of getting burned, as psoriasis has a tendency to develop on damaged skin. This can happen on an accidental cut, on an operation wound or on sunburnt skin, and is called the **Koebner phenomenon**, after the man who first recognized it. For a minority of psoriatic sufferers, sunlight aggravates rather than improves the condition.

Some psoriasis sufferers need a little more help than emollient ointments and sunlight. The usual additional creams and ointments prescribed contain tar, dithranol, and, for limited parts of the body, topical steroids (cortisone-containing creams, ointments and lotions). The modern way to use dithranol preparations is to apply them to the skin for only 15–30 minutes each day, either in the morning or just before bedtime. Most people spend this time in an old dressing gown, on which any staining from the ointment does not matter. The dithranol is then washed off in the bath or shower and normal clothes can be worn without the need for bandages, and without clothes becoming stained. This is a much more socially convenient way to control psoriasis than the treatments recommended a few years ago, which used messy and strange-smelling ointments that were applied under bandages under normal clothes through the day. A further recent development is the introduction of an ointment containing an active ingredient very similar to vitamin D, which appears to be effective, clean, odour-free, and non-staining (calcipotriol or Dovonex).

Most psoriasis sufferers can tolerate a few scaly patches on their back or other covered sites, but are embarrassed about patches on their face or hands. Other people can be unthinkingly unkind, and many assume that all skin disease is infectious. Visible psoriasis can be a problem in many occupations, particularly those that involve dealing with the public or handling food. Visits to the hairdresser can also pose problems as psoriasis sufferers can receive less than kind treatment from hairdressers who do not know that psoriasis can do no harm whatever to others. The Psoriasis Association may be able to provide a list of local hairdressers who are more understanding (for address see p. 143).

A small percentage of people with psoriasis have problems that are not controlled by treatment with creams, ointments, and exposure to either natural or artificial sunlight. In these cases further treatment is available in the form of tablets or injections. The general principle behind the oral psoriasis treatments is that they slow down the rate at which cells divide in the skin. However, they also reduce the rate at which cells divide in other parts of the body, including the bone marrow, where the blood-forming elements are made. Because of this, it is essential that the person receiving treatment has regular blood checks to make sure that they are producing sufficient red cells, white cells, and platelets, which are important in helping the blood to clot. In addition, it is essential that young women requiring this type of general treatment for psoriasis do not become pregnant, as these treatments could damage an unborn baby. Reliable contraception such as the oral contraceptive must be used concurrently with such treatments, and continued for a varying period of time after the treatment is stopped, depending on exactly which type of antipsoriatic treatment was given.

PUVA

An effective and commonly used treatment for those with severe psoriasis is **PUVA**. This involves taking a psoralen tablet by mouth and, 2 hours later, receiving treatment in a special cabinet fitted with tubes that emit ultraviolet radiation of the longer wavelength in the UVA range. This explains the name: Psoralen + UVA = PUVA. PUVA is effective at clearing psoriasis, and the sufferer can then change over to other methods as maintenance treatment to prevent recurrence. As with other treatments for severe psoriasis, PUVA cannot be used by young women who wish to add to their family, as psoralen could harm the developing fetus.

6.

Care of more mature skin

From the age of about 40 onwards, skin care is mainly directed towards preventing dryness. A dry skin is a wrinkled skin and wrinkles are generally associated with 'ageing', something most people would like to delay as long as possible.

Over the past 50 years modern medicine has made tremendous advances. Nowadays it is possible to replace damaged hearts and other organs, to provide treatment to take over the function of failed kidneys, and to treat diabetes with daily insulin injections. But we cannot replace the skin, so it makes very good sense to look after it as well as possible, and to begin this care early in life. This is particularly important now that in developed countries many of us can expect to live well into old age.

It is important to distinguish between what is inevitable, or **intrinsic ageing**, which we cannot prevent and must accept more or less gracefully according to our personality, and other features seen on the skin of older people that are partly preventable or can at least be delayed.

The skin on the face of a healthy 60-year-old (see Figure 18), shows some fine wrinkles, perhaps some deeper lines, a few broken veins on the cheeks, and some variation in the skin colour. By contrast, the skin on the buttocks is usually smooth, soft, and a uniform colour. What has caused the 'ageing' changes on the face, and why does the covered area look younger? The answer is exposure to sunlight, which causes '**photo-ageing**' that, unlike intrinsic ageing, can be at least partially prevented or delayed.

One of the best demonstrations of the importance of photo-ageing is a comparison of the skin of someone who has lived all their life in Northern Europe or the northern US with that of a relative of a similar age who emigrated to Australia or to the southern part of the United States early in life—the relative who emigrated will usually look older for their years because of the weathering and ageing effect of constant sunshine on the skin. In the Department of Dermatology at Glasgow University we almost

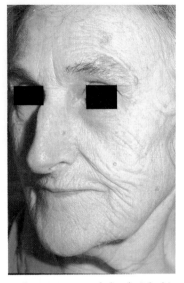

Figure 18 The normal appearance of the facial skin of an elderly individual. Much of this is photo-ageing, not intrinsic ageing.

always have a young dermatologist visiting us from Australia or New Zealand for a year as part of their training. Many of them comment on how very much younger-looking Glaswegians are than Australians or New Zealanders of the same age. So the frequently damp and grey climate of the United Kingdom does have some compensations in terms of protecting our skin against sun-induced damage.

GENERAL CARE OF DRIER SKIN

As we get older the sebaceous glands in the skin steadily slow down and become less active. The skin therefore becomes drier, partly due to a lack of the naturally-produced grease on the skin and partly because this sebum on the skin surface encourages the skin to attract and retain moisture from the surrounding atmosphere. The dryness is therefore due to a combination of lack of both water and sebum. This drying of the skin is accelerated by sun, wind, and a dry, centrally-heated or air-conditioned environment indoors. An additional but usually very temporary drying environment is the pressurized cabin of an aircraft. After a long flight, most people will notice that their skin is very dry for a day or two. This is because the pressurized atmosphere of the aircraft cabin has a very low humidity and literally sucks the moisture out of the skin. This can be partly compensated for by drinking plenty of water and fruit juice—not alcohol, which is dehydrating—and by using plenty of rich moisturizer before, during, and for a few days after the flight.

MINIMIZING MOISTURE LOSS FROM THE SKIN

The face

People who had a relatively oily or greasy skin as teenagers, and who may have suffered from acne, have the compensation that as they grow older their skin will often look younger for longer because they have had a greater regular output from their sebaceous glands. Those who had perfect 'normal' skin as teenagers will usually find on the other hand that their skin is looking drier earlier. The signs that skin is becoming a little more mature are the appearance of wrinkles at the sides of and under the eyes, very often around the mouth, and often on the neck. This is also frequently associated with a steady drying of the skin on the hands, particularly on the backs, and dryness, sometimes with fine scaling, of the shins of the lower legs, particularly during the winter months.

All these features are signs that the body's own naturally-produced lubrication—sebum—no longer offers enough protection against the environment and the daily skincare routine needs to be adapted to compensate. Any part of the skin that is habitually dry, feels tight after washing or has fine scaling needs some additional replacement of moisture. As far as the face is concerned, most women start by changing from soap and water to a non-drying cleansing cream or lotion. Provided this removes make-up and grime at the end of the day and leaves the skin feeling soft and comfortable, this is a sensible step and prevents the remaining production of the sebaceous glands on the face from being immediately washed away by soap and water. Similar cleansers can perfectly well be used by males, and men with a dry, tight or uncomfortable feeling skin should investigate the range of skin care products available in, for example, the Body Shop.

After cleansing, most older skins will benefit from the use of a moisturizing cream. Many moisturizing and emollient preparations are neither tinted nor scented and are therefore perfectly appropriate for use by both sexes. They are usually needed around the eyes and on the cheeks, as in contrast the so-called central panel of the face, the area that has most sebaceous glands, can supply its own lubrication for longer.

The rest of the body

As far as the rest of the skin is concerned, many people find that a bath additive or a moisturizing showering gel or lotion helps. A wide range of these bath and shower additives is available, aimed at both sexes, and most of them do the skin nothing but good. A few people may have an allergic contact dermatitis to either fragrances or to the lanolin that may be found in some bath additives and moisturizers. If this is the case, they should use alternative fragrance-free and lanolin-free preparations.

Often, only certain body sites, such as the shins or the elbows, are particularly dry. These areas can benefit from regular use of a simple hand cream or other emollient applied after a bath or shower. Most moisturizers work best if they are used after the skin has been washed and then gently patted dry, so that a little water is still visible.

It is especially important that outdoor people who enjoy activities such as golf, gardening, and walking, get into the habit of applying a moisturizing preparation to the skin every morning as part of their regular routine. Many of these preparations contain a built-in sun-screen, and even in northern Europe and the northern US it is worth using such a sun-screen during the summer months. Older people may spend more time on outdoor pursuits and if sensible care is not taken to avoid skin damage from sun exposure, the avoidable sun-induced or photo-ageing will be accelerated. A thin layer of a moisturizer containing a sun-screen applied every morning, and the use of a comfortable, shady hat if the weather is particularly sunny, are sensible approaches to keeping the skin of the face as good-looking as possible for as long as possible.

An outdoor hobby or occupation may involve being out-of-doors in all weathers in the winter months. Reading about sun-screens for such occupations may cause a smile or more likely a snort of disbelief. Remember, however, that strong winds lashing against the face can also cause weathering, the appearance of little dilated blood vessels on the cheeks, and chapping and soreness. In winter the use of a thicker, moisture-retaining preparation will protect the skin and prevent the biting winds from doing their worst.

Many older people keep the temperature of their homes relatively high as they feel the cold more, possibly because of a poor circulation and because they are less active than in the past. With efficient central heating and a small modern house or flat, it is important to be sure that the air is humidified. This can be done by simply putting bowls of water near the radiator, or rather more elegant humidifiers can be purchased and used. This is particularly important for older people who do not get out a lot and who spend most of their days in the one well-warmed room. The humidifier will also be good for any wooden furniture, and the piano if there is one—as a very dry environment is just as bad for the wood of antique furniture as it is for more mature skin.

All of these suggestions about humidifying the home for the good of the skin apply equally to the workplace. Many modern office buildings are over-heated and have low humidity. If a window can be opened, fresh air will help to counteract this damaging atmosphere.

MINOR SKIN CHANGES ASSOCIATED WITH INTRINSIC OR INEVITABLE AGEING

As we pass through our forties and fifties, a number of small changes may take place on the skin, even on parts that are normally covered up from sun exposure. Many of these changes are totally normal and benign and require no special attention.

Small cherry-red spots, very often only 1–2 mm in diameter, may develop on the trunk; several may appear at any one time. The medical name for these is **Campbell de Morgan spots**, after the individual who first described them. They are of no particular importance and are in no way any type of skin cancer or precancerous change in the skin. Unless they are causing problems they should be left alone.

Also very common are the small warty, slightly scaly, brown areas a little bit raised above the skin surface that appear on covered

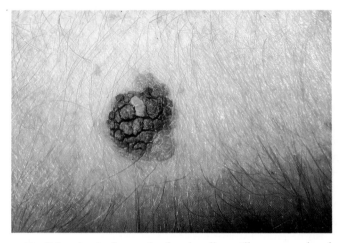

Figure 19 Seborrhoeic keratosis (basal cell papilloma or seborrhoeic wart). These are common, harmless marks, most frequently on the trunk, which are neither skin cancer nor a precursor of skin cancer.

and uncovered skin. There are several names for these: **seborrhoeic warts, seborrhoeic keratoses** and **basal cell papillomas** (Figure 19). They are a minor and unimportant overgrowth of the more superficial part of the skin, the epidermis. Although one of the names for these little changes is a seborrhoeic *wart*, they are not caused, as far as we are aware at present, by the wart virus. These little scaly lesions are usually quite easily kept under control by the regular gentle use of a loofah in the bath to remove any superficial scaling from their surface. If they give rise to discomfort or cosmetic embarrassment they can be easily removed, either by freezing or by the use of an electric needle to cauterize the area. Surgical excision and stitching are not usually required. They are not a form of skin cancer, nor do they turn into skin cancer.

A third minor change, usually found on facial skin in older people, is the appearance of little broken blood vessels or small capillaries. These are usually seen on the cheeks and nose of people who have always had a high colouring. Contrary to popular belief, they are not the result of years of heavy drinking of alcohol, and life-long teetotallers who have these little veins do not find jokes about them amusing! These are difficult to remove and, once developed, are best treated by a light covering of cosmetic. It is therefore best not to let them develop in the first place by protecting the skin from harsh weathers with a moisture cream and by not sitting too close to an open fire. Victorian ladies knew this, and positioned elegant little fire screens to protect their faces from the heat of the fire and preserve their alabaster complexion.

Women in this age range may also be concerned about a reddish brown, almost stain-like, mark on the side of the neck. The dermatological name for this is **berloque dermatitis**, and it is a result of applying perfume or toilet water to the sun-exposed skin of the neck. The sunlight and the perfume interact, and this discoloration is the result. The simple solution is to spray the perfume on to skin that is not exposed to light where it will not cause any discoloration.

CARE OF THE LEGS

As we become older, the skin of the lower leg becomes more fragile and cuts and grazes that healed rapidly in childhood now take much longer to heal over. This is partly because the blood supply to the skin of the lower leg has to work against gravity, pumping blood back up to the heart. It is therefore important to protect the legs against grazes from supermarket trolleys, minor gardening accidents, and nicks while shaving.

The lower legs are always a relatively dry area of body skin, even when young. In older people, either cold winter winds or a holiday in drying sunshine may cause dry, scaly, and even chapped skins. A rich body lotion will help prevent this, as will the habit of wearing warm stockings, tights, or trousers in the colder winter months.

VARICOSE VEINS

Varicose veins of the lower legs can also give rise to skin problems. Varicose veins are more common in women than men, and are usually more of a problem in those who are overweight. A common pattern is that mild varicose veins develop during a pregnancy, and have then become a little worse with subsequent pregnancies. Varicose veins not only look unsightly, but also make legs feel tired and heavy at the end of the day. Varicose veins can be recognized as thick veins which protrude from the skin's surface when the sufferer is upright, but almost disappear when lying horizontal. At the end of the day, the affected leg often feels uncomfortable and heavy.

Varicose veins frequently appear first on the skin over the inner surface of the ankle, the calf, and the thigh, and they are quite distinct from the little thread veins which do not protrude above the skin's surface and often appear on the thighs of women. These thread veins are a purely cosmetic problem, and although they can be obliterated by a simple cosmetic injection, this is not medically necessary.

As soon as early signs of varicose veins are seen, a doctor should be asked for help. A simple course of injections, bandaging, and regular walking exercise may be all that is required. Losing weight is also a very important part of curing varicose veins and preventing them deteriorating.

Surgery may be needed for more advanced varicose veins but many surgeons feel they cannot operate unless the sufferer loses some weight and promises to maintain a sensible weight after surgery. This is because the problem tends to return if the patient is significantly overweight. The type of surgery carried out will depend on the surgeon and on the severity of the problem. In some cases a number of cuts are made in the legs and perforating veins linking the deep and superficial veins of the legs are tied off. It may then be necessary to use support bandages or support stockings and to exercise. The success or failure of this particular operation often depends on what the individual does to help themselves in the week or two after surgery.

The particular skin problems associated with varicose veins are **stasis dermatitis** or **eczema**, and **varicose ulcers** (see Figure 20). If varicose veins are left untreated the area of skin on the inside of the ankle area may become red or even brown in colour, irritable, and itchy. This is varicose dermatitis, and is a sign that blood from the veins has leaked into the surrounding skin; a swollen vein will often be seen close to this area. If this vein is bumped and damaged, for example during a fall, it may break down completely and a stasis or varicose ulcer will result. Once formed, these are very difficult both to heal and then to keep healed, because the skin is already so badly damaged by the varicose veins themselves, and by the eczema.

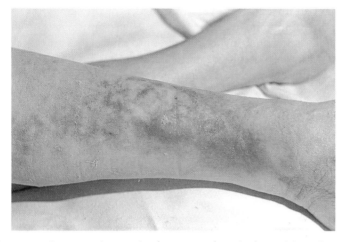

Figure 20 Severe varicose veins have caused stasis dermatitis and a very early ulcer on this leg.

The lower legs must be protected, overweight should be avoided, and the family doctor should be consulted about varicose vein treatment if necessary.

SKIN CARE AND THE VERY ELDERLY

Many households nowadays include an elderly relative. Skin care for the over-80s is directed at keeping the skin clean and comfortable, and replacing lost moisture. As long as the elderly person can manage a shower or, preferably a bath, the addition of a moisturizing bath oil is a good way to achieve this, although they make the surface of the bath greasy, which might cause the elderly person to slip when getting in or out of the bath. A mat in the bath and firm handrail will help prevent this.

If getting into the bath is no longer possible, a bed bath may be necessary. In many cases a district or practice nurse will call to help with this, but if there is no professional help available, the following advice may be useful.

Only attempt to wash one area—one arm or leg—at a time. Older people become chilled very quickly, so cover the rest of the body with a blanket or warm towel. Use a soapy face-cloth and rinse off all traces of soap very thoroughly, or the skin will become even drier and very irritable. Dry the skin gently but thoroughly and apply a moisturizing lotion, except to the flexures where talcum powder is more suitable. Be particularly careful with the skin of the back. If the old person is confined to bed, this skin will have to bear the weight of the body continuously. Keep it as clean, dry, and comfortable as possible, and either help the old person to move around the bed a little or turn them regularly. Lying on a sheepskin may also help. It is important to try to prevent this skin breaking down and causing bedsores because like leg ulcers, these are very difficult to heal once they develop.

If the elderly relative is either confined to bed or requires a wheelchair, the problems are even greater. The skin of the very elderly is thin and fragile, and will easily break down, causing a pressure sore that can cause continuous pain and discomfort. Healthy people are continuously moving slightly as they sit or lie, so that the skin over one area of the back or buttock area is not subjected to the weight of the entire body for any length of time. Elderly people, who perhaps have had a minor stroke, are not always able to do this. It is therefore vitally important to be sure that they sit or lie on a soft, dry surface, and that they are assisted to move around a little even at night. The skin of the weight-bearing areas should be checked daily if possible for any minor problems, and massaged to help the circulation.

CARE OF THE FEET

Many older people have chronic problems with their feet. These problems may relate partly to the skin and partly to underlying bony problems, often the end result of years of wearing ill-fitting footwear. Once bunions, corns, and callosities have developed, the problem of finding a comfortable shoe becomes even greater, and clearly the best long-term approach to this is prevention in the first place. Older people with foot problems should see a chiropodist regularly, and in the UK this can be arranged through the National Health Service. Be careful about amateur treatment of corns or other problems, as cuts and injuries to elderly feet heal very slowly because of the reduced efficiency of the circulation of the blood. Painful dry hacks may develop in colder weather, particularly on the heels. Prevent these by applying a generous application of rich hand cream to the area.

Poor circulation may lead to cold feet, and the desire to warm them quickly in hot water, using a hot water bottle, or by the fire. Rapid rewarming of cold feet can cause chilblains, so try to stop the feet becoming cold by wearing warm socks, if necessary bedsocks, and warm roomy winter boots. Remember that the best way of keeping the circulation moving briskly is by taking some exercise.

7.

Sun and the skin

The preceding chapters of this book have emphasized that too much exposure to both natural sunlight and artificial ultraviolet sources such as sun-beds and sun-lamps, is not good for the skin. This chapter explains this in more detail and offers advice on sensible sun exposure for all ages. Guidelines will be given to explain how sun-screen and sun-block preparations are graded and classified.

ULTRAVIOLET RADIATION

Figure 21 illustrates the relationship between ultraviolet radiation and the other types of non-ionizing radiation, such as natural light and infra-red radiation. It will be seen that ultraviolet radiation from the sun is divided into three different wavelengths—UVA, UVB, and UVC. The UVA waves are the longest and the UVC the shortest. Figure 22 shows the approximate penetration of UVA and UVB rays into the epidermis and dermis. UVB rays do not penetrate further than the basal layer of the epidermis, but UVA rays go much deeper than this—into the mid-dermis. This difference in penetration explains different long-term effects of UVA and UVB on the skin.

UV AND THE OZONE LAYER

At present, UVC is prevented from reaching the earth's surface by the ozone layer, and is not therefore a natural hazard. There is, however, concern that the loss of the protective layer of ozone above the earth's atmosphere will continue, and that in future more UVB might reach the earth. Ozone currently absorbs all UVC and a proportion of UVB from the sun's rays, but emission of chlorofluorocarbons (CFCs) from aerosols and other sources is destroying this protective ozone layer and will continue to do so if further national and international action is not taken. As it will take up to

nm	254	290	320	360	
X-rays		UVC	UVB	UVA	Visible light

At present no UVC reaches the earth's surface.
UVB is the main wavelength in natural sunlight.
UVA is the longer wavelength emitted by sunbeds.

Figure 21 The place of ultraviolet radiation in the electromagnetic spectrum.

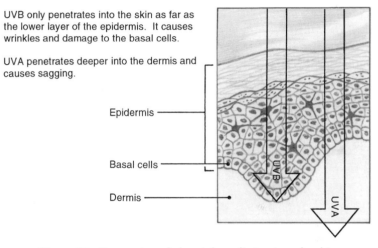

UVB only penetrates into the skin as far as the lower layer of the epidermis. It causes wrinkles and damage to the basal cells.

UVA penetrates deeper into the dermis and causes sagging.

Epidermis

Basal cells

Dermis

Figure 22   Penetration of ultraviolet radiation into the skin.

50 years or more for the ozone mantle to repair itself, this is currently regarded as a matter of major ecological importance. If more UVB rays were to reach the earth's surface they would contribute to sun-induced burning of the skin, would increase the risk of skin cancer, would cause damage to the eyes—producing cataracts in humans and animals—and would also cause extensive damage to plant systems.

UVA AND UVB

The main ultraviolet component of natural sunlight that does reach the earth's surface is UVB. This penetrates the epidermis and reaches the more superficial layer of the dermis—the papillary dermis. UVA is also present in sunlight and, in the early spring, a high proportion of natural sunlight in countries at latitudes 50 degrees or more north or south of the Equator (e.g. the more northern states of the US, the UK and New Zealand) is composed of UVA. As the summer develops, the proportion of UVA falls.

UVA is the main, but not the only, wavelength found in the long tubes in UVA sunbeds. The effects of UVA go deeper into the skin than those of UVB. A very simple rule of thumb is that chronic over-exposure to UVB causes wrinkles, chronic over-exposure to UVA causes sagging, and chronic over-exposure to both increases the risk of developing skin cancer. One of the important points of difference between UVB and UVA exposure is that acute over-exposure to UVB causes the redness and soreness recognized as sunburn. This is maximal 12–24 hours after the exposure has taken place, and is a useful warning that the skin should be protected for a few days until the redness has disappeared. In contrast, however, acute over-exposure to UVA may show no warning redness and even if a little pinkness develops, it takes up to 72 hours for this to show. So there is no immediate warning that the damaged skin has had an excess of UVA and needs protection for a day or two.

WHAT HAPPENS WHEN SKIN IS EXPOSED TO SUNLIGHT?

A number of biologically important events are triggered when skin is exposed to ultraviolet radiation. Short-lived structures called **free radicals**, which consist of a few atoms, are generated and, although these are very quickly destroyed by a number of scavenging systems in the skin, they do some damage. In addition, part of this is damage to DNA—deoxyribonucleic acid—the basic genetic building material of all living matter.

DNA makes proteins, which are the basic component of cells in the skin, muscle, blood vessels, and all other parts of our bodies. There are complex systems for repair of sun-damaged DNA but these are not inexhaustible, and cannot cope with excessive sun exposure over many years. Over time, therefore, faulty DNA is not corrected, and this in turn increases the risk of skin cancer. For many years during childhood and young adult life these repair and

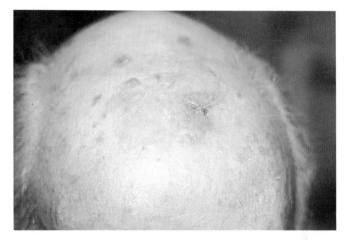

Figure 23 Actinic keratoses on the scalp. This is a sign that the skin in this area has had excessive sun exposure.

protection systems are adequate but, after a variable period of time, depending on inherited characteristics such as skin colour and also on external variables such as the age at which we receive sun exposure, its intensity and duration, these repair mechanisms fail to keep up with what is required.

When this happens rough scaly patches of skin—**actinic keratoses**—develop (see Figure 23), with irregular patches of brown colour—sometimes called age spots, liver spots or sunspots. These are often seen on the backs of the hands and other chronically sun-exposed parts of the body.

The underlying elasticity in the dermis is lost, although, paradoxically, a lot of material appears in among the dermal collagen and through the microscope, this looks very like elastic tissue. This dermal damage cause wrinkles if the damage is done by UVB, and sags if it has been caused by UVA—neither very desirable. Chronically sun-exposed skin tends also to look leathery and thickened because of the deposition of this elastic-tissue-like material.

While all of the changes described above might be accepted by the dedicated sunworshipper as worthwhile, the next stage in the gradual build-up of chronic sun-induced damage is the development of skin cancers, described in detail in Chapter 8. These are usually of the non-melanoma type—the basal cell cancers and squamous cell cancers. They are relatively easily cured by surgery but, once one develops, it is highly likely that more will follow. In Australia, where it is difficult to keep out of strong sunshine, two-thirds of the population currently develop some form of skin cancer during their lifetime. Because of this a very large proportion of that country's expenditure on health care is devoted to skin cancer treatment.

A large proportion of skin cancers can be avoided if simple precautions are taken. Most countries have had to come to terms with a limited budget for health care and each nation has had to decide how much it can afford to devote to health care and then what this money should be spent on. With ageing populations in the so-called developed countries, this is becoming increasingly difficult, but the volume of medical need could be reduced by personal decisions to reduce behaviour that is widely recognized to be detrimental to health—smoking and excessive sun-exposure are two obvious examples.

Before sun-induced skin damage reaches the stage of frank cancer it causes considerable discomfort, with dry itchy skin. Many elderly people suffer from this—the end result of a lifetime of summer sun-bathing and the cultivation of what has in the past been thought of as a desirable and fashionable tan. These people may well regret their past sun-exposure and the continuous discomfort their resulting dry skin gives them. Unfortunately, a lot of the sun-induced skin damage to this generation was done before the serious long-term effects of chronic sunlight exposure were fully recognized, even by experts, and certainly before the public were fully aware of the problem. Nowadays the problem is widely recognized and sensible preventive behaviour can and should be adopted at a young age.

A BRIEF HISTORY OF THE SUNTAN

Until the 1920s and 1930s, the fashion among the upper classes was to have a porcelain pale skin. Fashion decreed long skirts, sun bonnets and parasols. A tanned skin indicated that one had to perform manual outdoor work to earn a living, rather than employ servants. This vogue for a pale skin changed after the First World War, when young people from the towns discovered the pleasures of outdoor sports, such as walking and hiking. Before the 1920s these activities were available only to the wealthy few but the development of, for example, the youth hostel movement, meant that the countryside became more accessible to all. Associated with this switch to an increased interest in and enthusiasm for outdoor exercise, fashions for women changed. Skirts became shorter and shorts became acceptable sporting wear. Thus, skin that previously had rarely seen sunlight was exposed, and the resulting suntan was seen as an attractive and cosmetically desirable fashion accessory. It is said that in France the activities of Coco Chanel in promoting a tan on the Mediterranean beaches gave fashion-conscious women an important role model.

The important social change after the Second World War was the easier access of sunny foreign holidays for all, with the development of package holidays and cheaper air travel. Once again the result was to promote the social desirability of a suntan and the idea that it was necessary to return from a vacation several shades darker than on departure was generally accepted.

Meanwhile, in the medical world it was slowly being recognized that sun exposure was associated with skin cancer. It was only in 1950 that this was widely recognized, although from the beginning of this century a number of workers had suggested that sun exposure was at least one of the causes of skin cancer in both animals and men. This illustrates just how long it can take for experimental work in medicine to be widely accepted and fitted into existing clinical practice. Then, in the early 1960s, it was recognized in Queensland, Australia, that the number of people with skin cancer, melanoma in particular, was reaching epidemic proportions. This resulted in the start of the Queensland Melanoma Project, which aimed to warn the public of the risks of sun exposure and educate them to recognize early curable melanoma. Nearly 30 years on, it appears that the Project has partly succeeded in that melanomas in Queensland are at present thinner, and therefore more easily cured, than they were 30 years ago, although the number of people developing melanoma still increases every year. Surveys of the population in Queensland, and many other parts of the world, show that while many people in these areas know that too much sun increases the chances of developing skin cancer, there has, until very recently, been a great reluctance to change habits and ration sun exposure. The difference between knowledge that a behaviour is harmful and taking steps to change that behaviour is an important one—very well recognized in the field of health education. This is particularly important when the behaviour—in this case obviously sun exposure—is seen as giving pleasure.

For those who live in parts of the world with long dark winters and relatively short summers—Scotland, Scandinavia and the northern US states are good examples—it is very tempting on a fine sunny spring day to spend an afternoon sunbathing in the park or garden. It is difficult to accept, especially when young, that the damage done if the skin is red and burned at the end of such an afternoon is cumulative, and that an invisible 'clock' in the skin is recording the number of hours spent in this way. In cooler parts of the world no visible damage will show until around the age of 40, but in sunnier areas even 25-year-olds have visible and permanent sun damage.

In countries such as Australia and Hawaii, with intense year-round sunshine, whole populations do now recognize very well the problems that excessive sun exposure can cause. This is seen at its worst in the white-skinned Caucasians in these areas, but even those with darker skins are at some risk. In these countries, children are not sent outside to play on a sunny day but are brought inside to shady verandahs and playrooms. They are quick to learn that the best place in the playground is in the shade of the biggest tree, and that peeling sunburn on a Monday morning is not a sign of a good weekend but rather that damage has been done to the skin. As a result of this public education, which begins in primary schools in these countries, a much greater awareness of the dangers of excessive sun exposure has developed. Together with this awareness, there is also a detectable change in behaviour with regard to sun exposure. This is good news for those involved in health education, as it is widely recognized that it is relatively easy to spread information, but much more difficult to bring about a change in behaviour, even if that behaviour is clearly recognized as being undesirable, or even frankly dangerous.

BENEFITS OF SUN EXPOSURE

The benefits of sun exposure include the previously discussed feeling of well-being and relaxation that a sunny holiday or even a sunny afternoon brings. In today's busy, stressful world, this is very welcome, but much of this feeling of relaxation can be achieved by relaxing under a sun-umbrella or in partial shade, and it is not necessary to roast the skin to achieve a feeling of relaxation, indeed bad sunburn will cause a very unrelaxed feeling.

In addition, ultraviolet light affects not only the skin but also, via special receptors on the retinae of the eyes, the central nervous system. Sunlight exposure generally induces a feeling of relaxation and well-being, and the converse is seen in winter, when some people in countries with very little winter sunshine develop a type of depression called **seasonal affective disorder** or, more appropriately, SAD. This problem appears to be improved by exposure to bright light.

The skin can synthesize vitamin D and, in those whose diet is deficient in this vitamin, this source may be important in preventing rickets, a disease associated with softening of the bones. Those who eat a normal western diet will consume plenty of vitamin D and, even if there is concern about adequate intake of vitamin D, a period of only 15 minutes in the sun each day is all that is required to supplement the body's dietary vitamin D.

Therapeutic artificial sunlight is prescribed for certain skin diseases. For example psoriasis, some cases of eczema, and the rare problem of cutaneous lymphoma. In all these cases the dose of ultraviolet radiation is carefully recorded, and not allowed to exceed what is currently regarded as a safe upper limit.

COMMON SENSE ABOUT SUN-SCREENS

Over the past ten years the range of creams, gels, and lotions marketed as sun-screens has increased dramatically, and there is now a bewildering display. Most of the containers carry the letters SPF. This stands for Sun Protection Factor, and the number after the letters is an indication of the strength of the preparation. For example, a cream with an SPF of 7 means that the wearer can be in the sun for seven times longer than they could if they were not wearing the preparation before the skin becomes pink—the medical term is 'minimal erythema'. The exact times involved will vary according to the time of day and strength of the sun. For example, at midday, it might take only 15 minutes' sun exposure before the skin becomes pink, and an SPF 7 cream would extend this to 105 minutes. However, this only applies if the preparation is applied thickly enough in the first place, and if it is renewed every 2 hours or so, and more often after swimming.

UVB RADIATION

At present the SPF system applies only to UVB protection and, unfortunately, there are different methods of calculating the SPF number in the US and Europe. This means that an American SPF 10 cream does not have exactly the same protective effect on the skin as a European product with the same number. There are currently moves to correct this situation but, in the meantime, the best approach is to choose a range of products and to move up, or down, the SPFs within that range. Thus, a product with an SPF of 10 will always be weaker than the SPF 15 cream in the same product brand range. If switching between brands, it is good advice to start with a higher SPF preparation than is normally used and work down. The reason for this is that at present there is no requirement for manufacturers to have SPF claims of their products assessed independently, and studies carried out by dermatologists have shown striking and disturbing differences between the claimed and the actual SPF of a given product.

At present, the higher SPF numbers widely available are in the 15–25 range, although products are on sale in the US with SPFs of over 40. A moment's thought would suggest that few people actually need a preparation of SPF 40+–when would you ever want or need to be in the sun for 40 times as long as it took to go pink without the cream? If this took 15 minutes, which is possible in strong sunshine, this would mean that you were planning to stay in the same sunshine for 10 hours. Fortunately for our skin this is just not possible, even in very sunny areas, because the sun is only at its most powerful for 4–5 hours each day. Countries such as Australia do not allow manufacturers to advertise an SPF number of greater than 15. This is partly to stop pointless competition between manufacturers to produce ever higher SPF numbers, which members of the public, who do not fully understand what SPF means, will assume must be better. One of the reasons for trying to prevent this is that the higher concentrations of the sun-screening chemicals found in these very high SPF preparations are associated with a higher frequency of allergic reactions.

UVA RADIATION

The SPF ratings apply only to the protection the cream offers against UVB damage, as it is UVB that causes the immediate redness and burning that is used to calculate the SPF factor. There are at present no widely accepted scales by which UVA protection is measured, although a system of stars (the more stars the greater the UVA protection) is proposed for the UK. At present, all one can do is study the package and see if any information on UVA protection is offered. There is currently a lot of research on a standard for measuring effective UVA protection, and it is hoped that this situation will improve rapidly.

PROTECTION AGAINST UVA AND UVB

The chemicals in sun-screens that protect against UVA and UVB can be divided into those that absorb ultraviolet radiation and those that reflect it away. The absorbing chemicals include para-amino benzoic acid—PABA—cinnamates, and salicylates, which protect against UVB alone. Benzophenones protect against both UVB and UVA and are also chemical sun-screeners.

Reflecting sun-screens contain zinc oxide and titanium dioxide, and protect against both UVB and UVA. They include the fluorescent face paints that have made sun-screening fun and fashionable.

Whatever the agent in the sunscreen, there is very little firm information on the stability of the product, and whether or not last year's tube will still be effective this year. In general it is probably better to start afresh, unless there is an expiry date printed on the container.

WHICH SUN-SCREENS ARE BEST FOR THE SKIN?

The answer to this depends upon the skin type. Dermatologists divide the population into several skin types, based on the balance between tanning and burning in the sun:

Skin type 1.   Always burns—never ever tans; this is quite rare.
Skin type 2.   Usually burns at first. Tans slowly and with diffi-
               culty. This is a common skin type in the north of
               the Europe, and in Americans with British or Scan-
               dinavian ancestry.
Skin type 3.   Tans easily, burns rarely.
Skin type 4.   Tans easily, never burns. Rare in the UK but common
               in Mediterranean countries and in Americans of
               Italian, Spanish or Greek descent.
Skin type 5.   Indian or similar shade of brown skin.
Skin type 6.   Black Afrocaribbean skin.

The skin type does not change, so no amount of wishful thinking
or lying on the beach will turn a type 2 skin into a type 4 skin.
Although, in general, fair hair and blue eyes go with types 1 and 2,
this is not always true, as there are some dark-haired, but usually
blue-eyed, individuals who burn readily. Such people are often of
Welsh, Irish, or Scottish descent.

SKIN TYPES 1 AND 2

People with skin types 1 or 2 will *never* achieve a deep, golden tan
and will cause themselves a lot of discomfort, if not actual pain, and
their skin some damage, if they try to do this. The midday sun
should be avoided both at home and abroad, and a shady hat should
be worn. Clothing is an excellent sunscreen as long as it is closely
woven. A pure cotton T-shirt is a cool, comfortable, and fashionable sun-screen, but a cotton lace-knit cardigan may let a lot of
burning sunlight through to the skin, and may leave a very strange
pattern of sunburn.

A sun-screening preparation with an SPF of 10 or more should
be chosen, applied generously, and re-applied every 2 hours and
after swimming. Studies on how we use sun-screens indicate that,
having brought our preparations, we do not apply them thickly
enough. A preparation that also states that it protects against UVA
is even better for the skin than one of the same SPF with no such
information. One of the ingredients to look for on the side of the
packet when seeking UVA protection is **microfine titanium
dioxide**.

SKIN TYPES 3 AND 4

Those with skin types 3 and 4 can safely allow themselves more sun exposure, but again should avoid the noonday sun. They will require some sun-screen protection with an SPF of around 8.

SKIN TYPES 5 AND 6

Those born with a darker brown or black skin have a good in-built sunscreen, but even they may need to use a sunscreen in very strong sunshine. Preparations with SPFs of 4–6 are recommended.

MOISTURIZERS

Whatever the skin type and skin colour, most people notice that their skin is dry after a lot of sun exposure, so plenty of emollients and moisturizing creams are a good idea. After-sun preparations are generally good moisturizers, but the usual moisturizing preparation will be just as effective. The important point is to apply generous quantities of these preparations after a day on the beach and for a week or two after returning home.

TAN PLANS

From time to time, women's magazines publish rather complicated 'tan plans', with instructions on using a preparation with, for example, an SPF of 15 for 3 days, then one of 12 for 3 days, and so on. These routines are both complicated and expensive. An alternative approach is to buy an SPF 15 preparation, to use it generously, and to gradually extend the time spent in the sun rather than switch to another preparation. This is easy, safe, and less expensive.

As far as a best-buy is concerned, the important point is to buy a preparation that will be used. Many people do not like very sticky preparations, and lotions are often more acceptable than creams. Some people find that their skin stings for a few minutes after using preparations containing para-aminobenzoic acid (PABA). However, PABA-free preparations are available. Cost is not necessarily a guide and the dearest preparation is not necessarily the best. It is advisable to buy 2 or 3 relatively inexpensive preparations from the chemist in small quantities, to find which one is most suitable and then buy the most economical size available. Sun-screens can be expensive, but relative to the cost of a lost day of your holiday because bad sunburn keeps you indoors, they are really quite good value. They are usually cheaper in a regular chemist or drugstore than in a holiday resort, and the range is usually wider.

Sun-screening preparations aimed at special body sites are available. Many women prefer a creamier, perhaps tinted preparation for their face, and either this or the general sun-screen should be applied to the neck area. In many women, the neck shows sun-accelerated age changes earliest, because it is exposed as much as the skin of the face, but often does not receive the same cosmetic care.

Sun-screening lipsalves are useful for both sexes, particularly if there is a tendency to recurrent cold sores. For many people with this problem sun exposure is one of the triggers of a new attack, and use of the lip-salve will reduce the chances of this.

SUN-SCREENS AND SPORT

Skiers and sailors need to be particularly careful with the sun. The problem with both these sports is that there is a great deal of reflected ultraviolet radiation from snow or water, which may cause burns on unexpected areas, such as the under surface of the chin. Another reason for problems is that, although there is a lot of direct and reflected sun, the air temperature is often low and sun-screening may be forgotten until late in the afternoon or early evening, when the skin becomes pink and painful. A thick waterproof sun-screen with an SPF of 15 should be used, and renewed every 2 hours or so.

SUN-SCREENS AND EVERYDAY LIFE

It is important to realize that sun-screens may be needed in the back yard or garden and on holiday in cooler areas, not only in the tropics and the Mediterranean countries. Many people apparently believe that sun in the northern US and the UK is never strong enough to do any real damage. A walk around a park on a sunny spring public bank-holiday weekend looking at the pink and painful backs will soon convince you that this is just not so. Those of us who spend the winter in grey northern climates have skin that is particularly likely to burn in early spring sunshine, as it has not yet had a chance to 'harden up' after being covered all winter, and we are all glad to have an opportunity to be out of doors relaxing and enjoying the fine spring weather. By all means do this, but remember that the skin is particularly vulnerable at this time of year.

POLYMORPHIC LIGHT ERUPTION

This used to be a relatively rare problem but is now seen much more frequently. It consists of small, very itchy blisters on the light-exposed areas of skin, chiefly the face and hands. It mainly affects young females, and is thought to be triggered by UVA. It is most often seen in the early spring. One of the theories as to why it has become more common over the past 10 years is that the availability of good UVB screening sun-screens has increased the time spent in the sun because they protect against the early warning signs of UVB-induced sunburn. These sun-screens have not, until very recently, been effective at also screening out UVB. The result is more exposure to UVA than ever before and it is suggested that this has caused the upsurge in the number of people with polymorphic light eruption.

To avoid this, choose a sun-screen that protects against UVA as well as UVB. Useful, relatively new, preparations include Boots' Soltan 20 and Sun E45 with an SPF of 15 or 25. These have good UVB protection as well as UVA protection. At present, the UVA screen may make the skin look a little pale, but it is worth having.

SUN-SCREENS FOR MEN

Some men apparently feel reluctant to use sun-screens because they feel that they are a form of cosmetic rather than a general skin care product like soap, and that male skin does not need sunscreens. This is not true! Although male skin is thicker than female skin it is not protected from sunlight any better, and in fact many more men than women develop non-melanoma skin cancer.

The opposite is true for melanoma, as in many parts of the world more women than men develop melanoma but, once men develop melanoma, they do not respond as well as women to treatment. Sun-screens should therefore be used by men and there are plenty of clear, non-tinted, non-sticky preparations available, which most men prefer.

SUN-SCREENS AND CHILDREN

The skin of young children is particularly susceptible to sun damage—both immediate damage in the form of sunburn and damage that is not immediately visible but is remembered by the skin and that will perhaps become obvious in later life. This is very well-illustrated by the skin cancers seen in emigrants from countries with relatively little sunshine, such as British emigrants to Australia. Far higher numbers of those who were born in Australia develop all types of skin cancer than those who emigrated there as children. What happens to the skin in the sun even before about 10 years of age affects the chances of developing skin cancer as adults.

Small babies under the age of 6–9 months should be protected completely from the sun. They should lie in the shade or under a canopy in the pram. After this age, sun exposure should be rationed so that the child is never even slightly burned at the end of the day. A loose, comfortable cotton top and a sun-bonnet or sun-hat should be worn. There are sun-screens aimed specially at children's skin, usually with a high SPF. These should be used when the child is in direct sun, and should be re-applied after paddling or swimming.

The Australians have a slogan—Kids Cook Quick! It is a good reminder about how careful we should try to be with children's skin.

An American dermatologist working on the problem of skin cancer has calculated that if all Americans used a sun-screen with an SPF of 15 daily until the age of 18, then the incidence of the non-melanoma types of skin cancer could be reduced by 78%.

TEENAGERS AND SUN

Peer group pressure amongst teenagers may make it particularly difficult to persuade this age group that a suntan is not necessarily desirable. At this age thoughts of personal skin cancer are almost impossible, and even ageing seems to be something that happens only to other people. It is therefore very important to try to persuade opinion-makers among teenagers that a tan is not desirable. Once again the Australians are leading the way, with their campaigns aimed specifically at teenagers promoting a 'sun-smart' and 'sun-cool' pale, attractive, and fashionable image.

SUN-SCREENS AND OLDER PEOPLE

Many older people may think that this advice about sun-screens to prevent early ageing is a bit late for them, and that the damage is already done. However, this is not so. The message with regard to sun-screens and sun exposure is that it is never too late to change our ways, and that some sun-induced damage *can* actually be undone if sun exposure is rationed and sun-screens are used. Now that many people in Europe and North America are retiring early and embarking on 'third age' careers, hobbies, or other activities, this becomes steadily more important. An individual retiring at 60 years of age may well have 30 years of active life ahead of them, and may plan to travel and enjoy outdoor activities, such as gardening or golf more than ever. It is now possible to spend a large part of the winter months in a warmer climate, closer to the Equator, rather than coping with snow, frost, and fog in northern Europe, or the northern US states. This is fine, but a high SPF sun-screen should always be used on hands, face, and any other exposed areas at the start of the day, and should be carried throughout the day so that protection can be renewed.

Individuals on regular medication for medical problems, such as high blood pressure and minor heart problems, need to be particularly careful, as some drugs can sensitize the skin to the sun. A doctor will know which medicines are photosensitizing, and should be consulted particularly if an extended winter stay in a sunnier country is planned. It is possible that the amount of sun at home is not sufficient to cause problems but that a red, painful rash soon appears in a warmer climate. As it may be very important to continue the medication equally effective but non-photosensitizing alternatives should be investigated.

SUN EXPOSURE ADVICE FOR THOSE WHO HAVE ALREADY HAD SKIN CANCER

Individuals who have had a skin cancer of any kind are at an increased risk of developing further skin cancers. This can be a quite separate problem, not a reappearance of the first lesion. These people should think carefully about sun exposure and should plan their days sensibly and should seek shade indoors or under a sun-umbrella while the sun is at its highest. A broad-brimmed hat should be worn to protect the head and shoulders and a sun-screen with an SPF of 15 or higher should be used. It may also be a good idea to have an annual skin examination to detect signs of further problems early.

SUNBURN AND HOW TO DEAL WITH IT

If, despite all precautions, the skin becomes sunburned, plenty of soothing moisturizer applied to the skin and aspirin taken by mouth will help. Aspirin has a specific effect in reducing the causes of sunburn-induced inflammation, so is preferred to paracetamol (UK) or tylenol (US). A tepid bath with added bath oil may help. A homely and soothing remedy is ice-cold milk applied straight from the icebox or refrigerator on a compress made from a handkerchief.

Hydrocortisone cream or ointment, provided it is only used in small quantities and just for a day or two, is helpful. Other soothing remedies include aloe vera.

The inflamed and sore areas of skin should be protected from further damaging sunburn until the redness and any peeling that develops have settled. This sounds very obvious, but holiday beaches are often covered by people with sore, pink backs determinedly exposing these backs to more damage. Put simply, a tan that has to be suffered for, and sun-bathing that causes redness and discomfort, is just not worth having. The short-term results will be unattractive and the longer-term results will be early ageing and perhaps, in time, the more serious problem of skin cancer.

ARTIFICIAL TANS

Artificial or fake tan products are usually found close to the sun-screens on the chemist's shelf. These usually contain **dihydroxyace-tone**, which stains the entire upper layer of the epidermis brown. This is a simple dyeing effect and is not the result of stimulating the pigment-producing melanocytes. If applied smoothly and uni-formly the results can be quite convincing to the eye, but this dye does not protect from sunburn, and an additional sun-screen will be needed. The fake tans do not wear off evenly, and the areas of skin that lose the superficial layers of cells fastest are easy to spot. For example, the skin over the Achilles tendon—the main tendon at the back of the ankle—is constantly rubbed by shoes, so the fake tan wears off more rapidly than from the more protected skin in the hollows around the ankles.

SUN-BEDS AND SUN-LAMPS

If natural sunlight is to be handled with care, what about the artificial variety? Nowadays most sun-lamps and beds are fitted with tubes that emit predominantly ultraviolet A radiation. In the past, so-called health lamps that emitted UVB were used, but these have been withdrawn from sale for some years now because of concern over safety. Sun-beds using UVA tubes are on sale to the public and are used in hairdressers' salons or at sports centres and other public places. Most people who use these sunbeds are either seeking a year-round tan or wish to begin to develop a tan before their annual holiday. The UVB part of the ultraviolet radiation spectrum is most efficient at causing skin tanning and so more exposure is required for a UVA tan than for a UVB tan and fair-haired, pale-skinned individuals may find it very difficult to develop a tan using a UVA sun-bed, although some type 1 and type 2 skin does develop large and somewhat unsightly freckles after exposure on a UVA sunbed. These may take a long time to fade, if they fade at all.

There are many other skin problems associated with using a sun-bed, and a group of dermatologists in the UK have recently published a list of sun-bed related problems in the *British Medical*

Journal. This list includes skin fragility, blistering, large unattractive freckles, and the possibility of skin cancer. In addition, UVA can interact with some oral drugs and cause an uncomfortable rash; such drugs include water pills (diuretics), antirheumatics, and some antibiotics.

In summary, UVA sun-beds are not good for the skin and tan developed on a sun-bed, if such a tan develops at all, will only have the protection of a factor 2 or 3 SPF sun-cream when the skin is exposed to natural sunlight. If a sun-bed must be used, it should be for only one course of 10 30-minutes exposures annually, and goggles should *always* be worn, as the eyes can also be badly damaged by UVA. This also applies to the sun-beds and facial sun-lamps marketed for home-use. At present, some states in the US are introducing legislation to prevent under-age teenagers using sun-beds either at all, or without parental permission. This emphasizes that the concern about sun-beds is general, and not limited to a small number of anxious dermatologists.

In summary, treat the sun with respect. It is quite possible to enjoy an outdoor life and a holiday in a sunny climate without doing the skin any harm. Look carefully at the habits of those who live all the year round in sunny countries. The noonday siesta makes very good sense, as it prevents exposure at just the time of day when the sun's rays are most damaging—provided, of course, that the siesta is under an umbrella or shady tree, not cooking painfully on the beach in the full glare of the sun.

Wear comfortable cover-up clothes: a long-sleeved shirt, long cotton trousers, and a shady hat are extremely effective for adults. Babies should never be exposed to full sunshine; there should always be a canopy over the pram. Toddlers, and even older children, should wear sun-hats and should never be allowed to develop sunburn.

Sunburn at the end of a day out-of-doors is a sign that the skin has had excessive exposure and should be protected completely from the sun next day and until the redness has vanished. Once this has happened a higher SPF sun-screen should be used, and time in the sun should be reduced.

8.

Skin cancer

Skin cancer is the most common type of cancer in the world, although it causes relatively few deaths. It follows that *most skin cancers are curable, provided they are recognized and treated early.* It is therefore extremely important that everyone should be well-informed about the warning signs of early skin cancer, both on their own skin and on that of their relatives and friends. Treated early, most skin cancers need be no more of a problem than a minor blemish but, if neglected, the more serious types of skin cancer can spread via the blood vessels to other parts of the body, and can even cause death. This is almost always preventable if the cancer is treated early.

While skin cancer can develop at any age it becomes steadily more common with age. In a climate such as northern Europe or the northern US, it is rare under the age of 50, but in sunnier countries such as Australia, it is seen not uncommonly in those in their 30s.

There are three main types of skin cancer:

(1) basal cell cancer, or rodent ulcer, which affects the keratinocytes;
(2) squamous cell cancer, which also affects the keratinocytes;
(3) malignant melanoma—the least common but most serious type, which involves the melanocytes.

The main cause of all three types of skin cancer is excessive exposure to sunshine. People living in sunny countries, such as Australia, and Americans living in the sunbelt states, such as Arizona and New Mexico, are at greater risk earlier in life.

All three types of cancer are curable if treated early. Over the past 5 years in the UK, the USA, Australia, and other countries there has been an emphasis on producing information for the public to help people to recognize skin cancer—and melanoma in particular—when it is early and curable. The results to date show that women have read this information and acted on it, coming for medical help with earlier, more curable skin cancers, while men appear either not to have read the information or not to have taken as much notice of it. For this reason, I very much hope that men will read this section of this book.

THOSE AT GREATEST RISK OF SKIN CANCER

1. Caucasians, i.e. white-skinned.
2. Usually aged over 40, but may be younger in sunny climates.
3. Have usually spent a fair amount of time in a sunny climate, either born there, worked there, or on holiday.
4. Are most likely to develop non melanoma skin cancer on the face, or the hands.
5. May first notice rough, dry skin on the head and neck—a useful warning sign.
6. May also have flat brown marks, sometimes referred to as age spots or sunspots, on their skin at these sites.

BASAL CELL CANCER

Basal cell cancer (also called rodent ulcer or basal cell epithelioma) is usually seen on the central panel of the face—the skin around the inner corner of the eye, and the area around the nose are commonly affected (Figure 24). Basal cell cancer is less common beyond the head and neck area. The first sign of a basal cell cancer is a raised, slowly growing little bump or nodule, which often has a rather pearly or translucent look to it. Such bumps will usually grow very slowly and quite painlessly for 6 months or a year before relatives or friends notice it. As it gets larger, small blood vessels may be seen on the surface and, if it is not treated, it will in time break down and form an ulcer. If still untreated, these ulcers can become very large indeed, and can spread down under the skin causing a lot of destruction to cartilage and even to bone.

TREATMENT

On the suspicion of a basal cell cancer the family doctor should be consulted. He may reassure the patient that the problem is not a

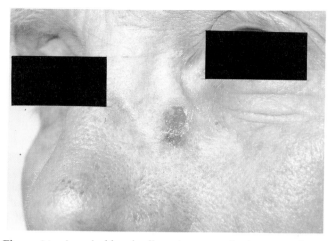

Figure 24   A typical basal cell carcinoma on the face, near the eye.

skin cancer but, if he feels that it may be a basal cell cancer he may arrange to remove it or make a referral to a specialist.

The hospital specialist will either arrange surgery or X-ray treatment—both are effective in completely curing basal cell cancer. The choice of treatment may depend on exactly where the rodent ulcer is and on the length of the waiting lists for the different types of treatment. Even if the choice of treatment is X-ray therapy, it is usual to remove a small sample of the suspected tumour first as a surgical biopsy, for examination under the microscope, to confirm the diagnosis. Before surgery, a local anaesthetic injection is given to make the area numb, and the small operation is usually carried out as an outpatient procedure or as day case surgery. The few stitches will be removed 5–10 days after the operation, leaving a small scar. The skin of the face heals particularly well because it has a very rich blood supply, and even quite large scars usually blend in very well with the natural lines on the face after a month or two. X-ray treatment involves attending a radiotherapy department, usually for two or three visits, and then keeping the skin clean and dry as the area heals.

Mohs surgery
If the skin cancer is close to a vital structure, such as an eye, for example, it is important to remove all the cancer cells but also

highly desirable to leave as much normal skin as possible. In this situation treatment may be by a special surgical technique known as **Mohs surgery**, named after Dr Fred Mohs, of Wisconsin, who developed the method when treating farmers from the American prairies with badly sun-damaged skin. This technique involves removing what the doctor hopes is all the skin cancer, and then immediately examining this under the microscope to see that the cancer has been completely removed. If not, more skin is cut away, while still using the same anaesthetic. This method takes longer because the samples removed have to be repeatedly examined under the microscope but, at the end of the operation, everything that needs to be done has been completed during one hospital visit. The Mohs technique is not needed for the great majority of skin cancer operations because as we get older there is plenty of loose skin on the face, and a skilful surgeon can often remove wrinkles or part of a double chin as an unexpected bonus during skin cancer surgery. It is, however, very useful for basal cell cancers in the central panel of the face and for basal and squamous cell cancers near the eye, where it is important to retain as much normal tissue as possible.

FOLLOW-UP

After any kind of surgery, and after X-ray treatment for skin cancer, it is necessary to attend either the family doctor or the hospital for regular check-ups. This is to make sure that the original problem has been completely eliminated and also because once one skin cancer has developed, there is a slightly increased risk of developing a second. A really good look at the skin in a mirror before the follow-up appointment is helpful, and the doctor's attention can be drawn to any new or changing mark or bump.

Some people with elderly relatives, perhaps over the age of 80, who have what they think may be a basal cell carcinoma may feel that it is 'unkind' or unjustified to seek treatment because of their relative's advanced age, and decide just to ignore the problem. Nowadays minor operations are very safe procedures and age itself should never be a bar to treatment; a healthy 80-year-old may well become a healthy 90-year-old. The family doctor should therefore be told of any changes on an older relative's skin, and will explain what would be involved in treatment.

SQUAMOUS CELL CANCER

This type of skin cancer is about a quarter as common as basal cell cancer. It usually develops on the skin of the head and neck, or on the back of the hands. Of the three types of skin cancer, this is the variety most clearly associated with constant exposure to sunlight over a lifetime.

The effect of sun exposure on the skin is both permanent and cumulative, and each 2-week holiday in a sunny country is 'remembered' by the epidermal cells. After 50 or 60 years this cumulative effects is very obvious. Thus, the effect of sun exposure is quite different to that of taking a drug, such as aspirin, where all traces are washed away within 24–48 hours, and a second dose at this time has just the same effect as starting afresh.

A common early warning sign that a person is at increased risk of developing squamous cell cancer is the appearance of small slightly raised, rough areas on the skin surface. These are **actinic keratoses** and it is usual to develop several of these, not just one. They do not brush or rub off easily, and may slowly expand (see Figure 23). Men may find them a particular nuisance while shaving, as they are easily nicked by the razor, causing bleeding. The good news is that they are reversible. If the skin on which these actinic keratoses have developed is protected from sunlight some will disappear over a period of about a year or so. If, however, the skin continues to be exposed to the sun, in time a squamous cell cancer may develop on or near these actinic keratoses.

A squamous cell carcinoma is usually recognizable because it is a raised, solid bump, which grows relatively quickly, perhaps doubling in size over 6 months or so (see Figure 25). It may adhere to the deeper structures in the skin, so that the skin cannot be made to slide easily over the underlying muscles and tendons in the usual way.

TREATMENT

Once again it should be stressed that any new growing or changing mark or bump on the skin should be shown to a doctor. He or she may cut a tiny piece out of a suspected squamous cell carcinoma— a biopsy—and, once this has been examined down the microscope

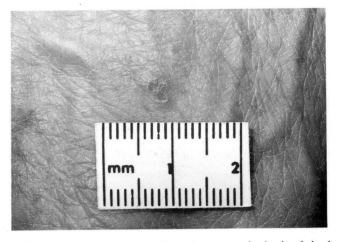

Figure 25 An early squamous cell carcinoma on the back of the hand. This may have developed from an actinic keratosis.

and the diagnosis confirmed, decide on the best treatment. Again this may be either surgery or X-ray treatment. As with basal cell cancer, a local anaesthetic is given before surgery and the cancer is then cut away, usually with a scalpel but sometimes by a high intensity cutting laser beam.

One of the advantages of laser surgery is that there is very little bleeding, so it is easier for the surgeon to see the exact area they are removing. However, because the laser beam seals off blood vessels, surgical wounds caused by a laser can take longer than usual to heal. Thus, laser surgery is not necessarily better in every way than conventional surgery, and the doctor will decide which method to use depending on where on the skin the growth is, what equipment is available, and other individual details of the case.

This type of surgery may be carried out by a family doctor, if they have had the appropriate additional training; by a dermatologist, who nowadays is required to attend special courses on skin surgery during training; or by a surgeon or plastic surgeon.

Stitches are removed 5–10 days after surgery. In addition, there will usually be some more deeply situated stitches under the skin, which are not removed. The material used for these deep stitches is designed to be absorbed, and they give the wound extra strength while healing takes place. Occasionally one or two of these stitches work their way to the skin surface, and may appear through the scar. This is not a reason for concern, nor a sign that a stitch was not removed at the correct time. It will take 3–4 months for the scar to become fully healed and strong, and even longer for the red appearance of a new scar to settle down to the usual skin colour and blend in with the surrounding normal skin.

FOLLOW-UP

Medical check-ups are necessary to ensure that the scar is healing as expected, and thereafter at regular intervals to ensure that there are no further problems with this area, and also to examine the rest of the skin in case a second squamous cell cancer develops. Once again, the affected person can check their own skin and draw the doctor's attention to anything that is new or has changed since their last visit. This is particularly important if the same doctor is not seen at every visit.

MALIGNANT MELANOMA

Malignant melanoma develops from the pigment-producing melan-ocytes. It is the least common of the three types of skin cancer but is responsible for most of the deaths from skin cancer. This is because the cancer cells developing from melanocytes—the malig-nant melanoma cells—are more likely to spread from the skin through the blood vessels and the lymphatic vessels to other parts of the body than are the cells involved in basal cell and squamous cell cancer. Once these malignant melanoma cells have spread, they can settle in any part of the body and continue to grow. For this reason it is particularly important to be able to recognize what could be an early malignant melanoma and have it treated when it is just starting to grow and is all still contained within the epidermis and higher part of the dermis. If treatment is carried out at this stage the prospects for cure are very good, and much better than for many other cancers, such as those of the breasts and lung.

Malignant melanoma usually starts as a growing and changing brown mark on the skin; there are four main types:

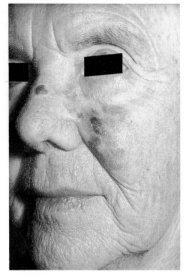

Figure 26   Lentigo maligna melanoma on the face of an elderly person.

1. The **lentigo maligna melanoma** most common on older faces.
2. The **superficial spreading melanoma**, most common on womens' legs and men's backs.
3. The **nodular melanoma**, a rapidly growing lump or bump found anywhere on the skin.
4. **Acral melanoma**—the rarest type in white-skinned people, found mainly on the soles of the feet.

Lentigo maligna melanoma

This melanoma is usually seen on older skin. It is most common on the face and may start as a slowly growing, irregular flat brown mark—a lentigo maligna—on the cheek (see Figure 26). After a year or two, if treatment is not carried out, a raised bumpy area may develop on this flat mark. Once it becomes raised and lumpy it is called a lentigo maligna melanoma. If this description is familiar as something seen regularly in the mirror, or on the face of a relative or friend, seek medical advice, or persuade the relative or friend to do the same. The British tend to be very reserved about such personal matters and are surprisingly reluctant to draw other peoples' attention to what could be a serious and even life-threatening problem on their skin. Studies from America show that Americans are better at encouraging others to seek early medical advice for possible skin cancer on exposed sites such as the face and arms.

Lentigo maligna melanoma is usually treated by surgery, but can also be treated by X-ray therapy. Even if the area of skin involved on the face is quite large, it is still likely that surgery can be carried out without the need for skin grafts and as a day case. The skin on the face of older people is usually lax and loose so there is plenty 'spare'. For this reason a skin graft is not often needed, as the extra skin can be moved around to fill the gap left by removal of the growth.

Superficial spreading melanoma

This is the most common type of melanoma. Melanomas are very rare indeed in children but do develop in young adults, although the most common age for developing melanoma in the UK is in the mid 50s. Here the evidence indicates that the relationship with sunlight is different to that seen with lentigo maligna melanoma and basal and squamous cell cancer, where the important factor appears to be the total time spent in the sun over a lifetime. In contrast, superficial spreading melanoma usually occurs in skin that has not been constantly exposed to the sun throughout the years but is subjected to intense intermittent sun exposure. This is exactly the situation where someone who spends most of their days indoors at home or in an office job goes on holiday somewhere hot and works hard at coming home with a deep suntan. Intensive basting on a sunny beach can result in the skin being exposed to as much sun in 2 weeks of holiday as it is for the whole of the rest of the year put together. This type of intense exposure of white skin to sun makes superficial spreading melanoma more likely, particularly if, in addition the skin is allowed to become badly sunburned. People at greater than average risk of this type of melanoma are those with a large number of moles, who may also have lots of freckles, and who may have some larger than average moles—greater than 5 mm in diameter, which cannot be covered by the blunt end of a pencil.

Early superficial spreading melanoma is usually seen as a new or growing brown mark that looks a little different from the moles or freckles around it. It looks different because it is growing or changing, and because it has an irregular outline, and is not a

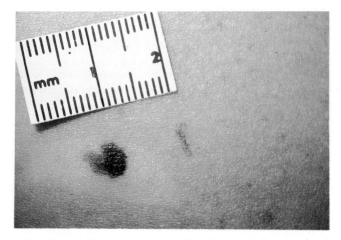

Figure 27   Superficial spreading type of malignant melanoma on the calf of a woman.

smooth circular or oval shape like most non-cancerous moles. It may also have different shades of brown in it, while normal, non-cancerous moles or freckles are all one shade.

Early melanoma is usually first recognizable when it is about 0.6 cm in diameter (Figure 27).

The most likely place for women to have melanoma is on the lower leg between the knee and the ankle; men are most likely to have it on the back. It is, of course, very difficult to notice a new or changing brown mark on your back, and melanomas on this site are usually first noticed by a friend or relative.

Melanomas may develop on what was previously normal skin, on a mole that developed during the teenage years, or on a mole that has been present either since birth or early childhood. These moles should not normally change at all and if any change is noticed, a doctor should be consulted.

Nodular melanoma

This type of melanoma appears as a fairly rapidly growing bump. It may be pink or red rather than brown, because the numbers of cancerous melanocytes are *multiplying* too rapidly to produce any brown melanin pigment (Figure 28). Sometimes, however, they have a thin brown rim of pigment. Nodular melanomas are more

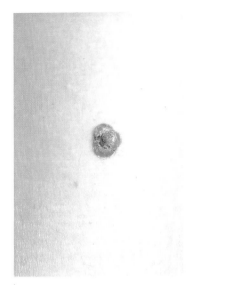

Figure 28 A nodular malignant melanoma on the thigh. Any rapidly growing lump or bump on the skin should always be shown to the family doctor.

common on older than younger skin and can develop anywhere on the body. Once again the important warning sign is *change*. A doctor should be consulted without delay if a new or growing lump, bump or brown mark is noticed anywhere on the skin, or if a mole or birthmark begins to look or feel different.

This, of course, means that you need to know what was there in the first place. It is a good idea to have a thorough look at your body from top to toe in a warm room using a full length mirror and also a hand mirror so that you can see your back. Make a note of anything bigger than about 1 cm, and look at yourself in this way again every 3–6 months. By doing this, you will become familiar with the minor blemishes and moles that are a part of you and that do not change. You will be quick to spot anything that is changing or behaving differently to the rest of your skin.

Acral melanoma

Acral melanomas are rare on white-skinned people, being more common on Asian skin. They appear as a growing, changing brown mark on the sole of the foot. A variant of acral melanoma also occurs under the nails of both the fingers and the toes. A sore area around a nail, which is not obviously an ingrowing toenail and refuses to heal, should be shown to a doctor. Many people who develop melanoma under a nail believe that the problem began with an injury, for example from a splinter or a rose thorn, but it is probable that this injury drew their attention to something that was there already rather than was the actual cause of it.

TREATMENT

Treatment of superficial spreading melanoma, nodular melanoma and acral melanoma depends on how far the melanoma has grown downwards into the dermis. This is calculated by looking down the microscope and measuring, in millimetres, the distance between the deepest melanoma cells in the dermis and the granular layer in the most superficial part of the epidermis. If this distance is 1 mm or less, all that usually needs to be taken away is a margin of 1 cm of normal-looking skin around the melanoma. In many parts of the body the edges of this wound can be brought together without the need for a skin graft, but the scar line is always longer than expected. A rough rule of thumb is that the scar will be three times as long as the length of the mark that was on the skin.

If the melanoma has grown deeper than 1 mm into the skin, a wider margin of normal-looking skin will need to be removed, and the surgeon will also need to take away more deep tissue. This means that a skin graft may be needed, usually taken from the thigh area. This area will be quite painful for a few days after removal of the graft because a lot of nerve endings will have been irritated. In contrast, the area where the melanoma was will usually be almost pain-free. Many people are surprised when the dressing over this area is removed, to see the skin graft apparently lying over a shallow hole. However, in about 6 months this area will have filled out and will look very much better. In the meantime, if the patient is a woman and the problem is on the leg, as is usually the case, the area can be temporarily camouflaged with thick tights or trousers.

FOLLOW-UP

After melanoma surgery, regular follow-up visits are necessary to make sure that the area is healing well and that there is no sign of the melanoma recurring. These visits may be quite frequent at first and then gradually extend to once every 3 or 6 months. It is a good idea to ask the doctor at these follow-up visits what exactly they are looking for. They are usually checking to see that there is no problem in the lymph glands in the armpit area, or the neck or the groin, as well as looking carefully at the skin around the scar. Knowing this will help prevent needless worry about other totally innocent and unrelated changes on the skin, and will also enable you to contact the specialist immediately if anything serious does develop.

This chapter on skin cancer is not meant to be depressing or alarming. Skin cancer is the type of cancer we are most likely to develop, particularly as we get older. A large proportion of skin cancers can be prevented and, if not prevented, they are curable if recognized and treated when at an early stage of development. Many people who have recently developed skin cancer in the UK have commented to us on how little information they felt was generally available about such a very common problem, compared with, for example, information on breast cancer. Such knowledge can be literally life-saving. Forewarned is forearmed.

9.

Cosmetics—myths or miracles?

Many different types and brands of cosmetics are available. The range of preparations and the claims made for them can give the impression that, provided money is no object, it is perfectly possible to obtain or retain a smooth, perfect, blemish-free, wrinkle-free, uniformly coloured skin throughout life. While some of the claims for new preparations may be justified, it is important to remember that the cosmetic industry is not controlled by the same type of code of practice that applies to the pharmaceutical industry for drugs, and that some of the claims made in advertisements may be based on very flimsy evidence.

Before a topical cream or ointment containing an active drug can be marketed as a medical product, a controlled trial comparing the new preparation with the best treatment currently available is carried out. Furthermore, this is done in what is called a '**double-blind**' setting, in which neither the person using the new preparation, nor the doctor supervising its use, knows whether the cream being applied is the new improved or the older established version until after the experiment. The equivalent of this in the cosmetic industry would be to take each new moisturizer and compare it with a recent competitor. This is occasionally done by the consumer watch-dog bodies, often with unexpected results but, for obvious reasons, is not carried out by the cosmetic houses themselves. This means that claims that laboratory tests 'show a significant improvement in 14 days' must be assessed thoughtfully by the purchaser.

Women vary in their attitude to cosmetics. Some feel little need for either skin care or decorative cosmetics and others spend a great deal of time, trouble and money on expensive preparations in both categories and feel 'undressed' without make-up. This chapter is aimed at people between these extremes, who wish to know if there are modern preparations whose sometimes dramatic claims may be justified, and who wish to delay signs of ageing and maintain a youthful and attractive appearance but without too much time or expense.

Preparations sold by the cosmetic houses fall into two main categories—skin care preparations and decorative or make-up preparations. The latter are very much a matter of individual taste. At present, however, there is a tendency for the distinction between the two to become very blurred, for example, tinted foundations, which have moisturizer or sunscreen added.

The official difference between cosmetic skin care preparations and a topical medicine, which is applied to the skin and at present in the UK usually requires a doctor's prescription, is that cosmetics, by definition, do not 'affect the body's structure or function.' In practice this means that they do not penetrate beyond the lower layers of the epidermis. In other words, if any cosmetic claims to be going deeper than the basal layer of the epidermis then in many countries around the world it is classified as a medicine or drug, and requires a prescription. It is therefore important to look with a slightly critical eye at some of the more dramatic claims made for modern cosmetics, particularly if they claim to do a lot of good to the deeper layers of the skin. This usually means the cells in the deeper part of the epidermis, and cannot or should not refer to an effect on the underlying dermis. However, this division between cosmetics and drugs or medicines acting on the skin is steadily becoming more blurred as newer ingredients are added to cosmetic to enhance their penetrating powers. It has been suggested that we may need to devise a new name for products that are more than cosmetics but less than drugs—the word 'cosmeceutics' has been proposed.

Cosmetics of the adornment or make-up category will not be discussed further, other than to emphasize that people can, and do develop, allergies to 'natural products'. Many people seem to believe that because a product is made from herbs or other natural substances they cannot develop an allergic contact dermatitis to it; unfortunately, this is not so. For example, it is possible to develop an allergic reaction to carrot oil; and lanolin, often thought of as a safe natural product is quite a common cause of allergies. So-called hypo-allergenic cosmetics are helpful but, unless the exact allergenic ingredient is known, and the ingredients of the cosmetic can be found out from the manufacturer, or preferably from a list of contents printed on the side of the bottle, it cannot be assumed that all hypo-allergenic products are suitable for all individuals with an allergy problem. Additional assistance may be required and advice from a dermatologist with an interest in this field is useful. At present in Europe there is an active campaign for full ingredient-labelling on all cosmetics, as has been law in the US for some years. This is necessary for consumer protection, and will make life much easier for those with allergies.

SKIN CARE PREPARATIONS

In general, skin care preparations are divided by the cosmetic industry into:

1. cleansers;
2. toners;
3. moisturizers;
4. special ingredients that, in the words of the cosmetic houses, 'nourish' the skin.

My personal preference would be to divide skin care into cleansing, moisturizing and sun-screening—as the evidence for the need for 'toning' is slim, and the value of sun avoidance is well illustrated and has been discussed in Chapter 7.

CLEANSING AGENTS

Soaps

Cleansing preparations can be divided into simple soap, cleansing bars, cleansers composed of water-in-oil or oil-in-water emulsions, and cleansing creams. Ordinary toilet soap is more alkaline and less acidic than the skin. The term pH is used to describe the acidity to alkalinity of the skin; a pH of 7 is neutral. Most soaps are alkaline rather than acid and have pH value or number higher than 7. There is, in fact, no dermatological evidence to show that a soap of an alkaline pH applied to the skin causes any damage, but a common belief has grown up that soap with a pH closer to that of our skin is in some way better for the skin.

It is best to trust your own judgement and the evidence of your own skin here. The alkaline pH soaps are generally the more common white or pastel-coloured bars we recognize as toilet soap, and if these remove dirt and grime effectively from the skin, and also remove such make-up as you choose to wear, without causing dryness, a feeling of tightness or any scaling of the skin, then there is clearly no need to look elsewhere.

The natural pH soaps are usually those that have a high glycerine content and are transparent. These are often very pleasant to use and may leave the skin feeling slightly smoother than an alkaline pH soap, possibly because of their high glycerine content rather than because of any pH difference. They are usually a little more expensive weight for weight than classic soap, but if they make the skin feel smooth and comfortable the extra expense may be worthwhile. One disadvantage, however, is that if left sitting in a pool of water they dissolve away remarkably rapidly.

Both men and women can suffer from contact dermatitis to fragrance. As mentioned before (see p. 64), fragrance does not mean just perfume, toilet water and after-shave. Fragrance and perfumes are added to many preparations that are used on the skin, and also even to some foods. Soaps often contain added fragrances and people with contact dermatitis because of a certain perfume, should use an unscented soap (for example Simple soap) to see if this makes their skin more comfortable. The lower pH, transparent glycerine soaps very often contain added fragrances, so they will not be appropriate for this particular problem.

A small range of specialist soaps contain either a deodorant or an antibacterial agent. These antibacterial soaps are often advertised for use by individuals with acne, particularly teenagers. However, soap is only in contact with the skin for a short period of time, so it cannot have a long-lasting effect. In general, if a deodorant or an antibacterial preparation is required, it is better to cleanse the skin with normal soap and then to use the appropriate tailor-made deodorant or antiseptic preparation.

Whatever type of soap is used on the face and body, it is important to rinse all traces of it away after cleansing. This is particularly important around the hair-line and under rings. People caring for elderly relatives who cannot get into the bath or shower should also ensure that no soap remains on the body after a bed-bath. If soap is left on the skin, the skin will become dry and irritated. Plenty of tepid water should be used to rinse off any remaining soap.

Other cleansing preparations

A wide range of cleansing preparations other than soap is available. These range from the cleansing preparations marketed for use on infant skin to the expensive cleansing creams and lotions aimed mainly at older female facial skin. Most of these preparations are pleasant to use but probably not essential if the skin responds well to soap. If, however, the skin is dry and tight after washing, or if a baby's skin becomes pink and sore after the use of soap, it is probably worthwhile changing over to one of the specific cleansing preparations. If an oil-based make-up is regularly used, a cleansing cream or lotion is necessary to remove all traces of the make-up from the skin, and a specialist cleansing preparation will be needed to remove eye make-up. This is particularly important because vigorous rubbing and scrubbing with soap around the eyes will not remove modern eye make-up, and will cause stretching of the delicate skin in this area, which will encourage development of lines and wrinkles.

Some cleansing lotions are designed to be applied to the skin and then removed with tissues or cotton wool, others are designed to be applied to the skin, rubbed up into a lather, and then rinsed off with water. This latter range is usually aimed at younger, oilier, teenage skin and may be very effective in this age range. By and large, however, they remove a high proportion of the surface lipid or grease from the skin, and are therefore less appropriate for older skin, as they may leave it feeling tight, stretched and uncomfortable.

Older skin usually benefits from a cleansing lotion that is wiped off. These work by forming a mixture or emulsion of the cleansing agent, residual make-up, and grime, which is all swept away on a tissue. It is easy to test their efficacy by applying a fresh white tissue to cleansed skin and examining it carefully for residual grime or makeup. The skin should not be stretched or pulled when using a tissue to remove cleanser. Water may, of course, be splashed on the skin after this, but these products do not foam up with water in the same way as the preparations aimed at younger skin. Some older people prefer to use a heavier cleansing cream, known in the past as cold cream and if this makes the skin feel clean and comfortable this should be used.

One of the questions on which many people would like advice is whether or not it is worthwhile paying more for an up-market product. In the case of cleansers, there is probably little reason to purchase an expensive preparation because the basic ingredients will be the same as in the cheaper products and the price will reflect the name of the cosmetic house or the packaging. I would recommend small sizes of the cheaper cleansers, possibly own brands from the large chemists and, once you have found a comfortable and effective preparation for your skin, to buy a large size and use it faithfully, at least every night, and possibly also in the morning.

However, remember that skin can develop an allergy to any of the components of any cosmetic. If you develop a reaction to a particular cosmetic, try an alternative that is both lanolin- and fragrance-free. Many of the large cosmetic houses make a low allergy range, or a range aimed specifically at sensitive skin. These are not all identical, so you may have to experiment to find which of these ranges is most suitable.

At the time of writing, dermatologists in the UK are campaigning to have the ingredients in cosmetics clearly labelled on the container as they are by law in the US. It would then be possible to avoid making expensive and painful mistakes, by selecting products that you know are free of the particular ingredient to which you have an allergy. This will be of particular value when a well-established cosmetic product is reformulated, and a new constituent that may cause problems for some users is introduced. It is always difficult to identify the culprit in contact dermatitis, particularly when the sufferer has used nothing new on their skin. Information on new ingredients added to well-liked favourite preparations would help to solve the problem more rapidly.

ASTRINGENTS AND TONERS

The second range of skin care preparations advertized by the cosmetic industry are the astringents or skin toners. The purpose of this range is stated removal of the last traces of cleansing agent, natural oil, and grease from the skin. The stronger astringent preparations, aimed at younger teenage skin, often contain alcohol and can be very drying indeed. They are said to 'tone' the skin and to help to 'close open pores'. Open pores are in fact slightly enlarged openings of the pilosebaceous (hair) follicles on the skin surface. (see p. 7). It is through these pores that sebum (grease) trickles to the skin surface. Many teenagers have some rather

enlarged-looking pilosebaceous openings on their facial skin, particularly on the cheeks close to the nose. There is to my knowledge
no proven evidence that astringents and alcohol will help to close
these pores, but if the skin feels more comfortable and less greasy
after the use of an astringent preparation, it will do it no harm.
Astringents can, however, be harsh to older skin, stripping it of all
traces of natural grease and lubrication, leaving it tight, shiny, and
uncomfortable. If patted on very vigorously over the cheeks, it can
result in the permanent appearance of small dilated blood vessels.
These can also result from spending a lot of time out-of-doors in
harsh weather.

Astringent preparations aimed at older people are often described
as skin toners. They may contain natural-sounding ingredients,
such as orange-flower water or witchhazel, and may be labelled
alcohol-free. If the skin feels fresh and comfortable after their use,
they do no harm. I am not, however, aware of any evidence to
show that they are in any way necessary for the skin's good health.

The equivalent of astringents for men are after-shave toners and
fresheners. These also have a drying effect on the skin, and many
are quite heavily perfumed. They are not recommended for use on
dry skin, and some of the fragrances used in after-shaves can be the
cause of troublesome allergic reactions, particularly if the skin is
exposed to strong sunlight.

MOISTURIZERS

The third main category of skin care cosmetics are moisturizers and
nourishing preparations. There is a very wide range both of
products, and of prices. At the lower end of the scale are the light
moisturizing lotions, which are generally inexpensive and often
aimed at both sexes and a wide age-range. These can be used not
just on the face but on any other part of the body, and may be non-
perfumed and non-coloured. Preparations such as Neutrogena
moisturizer come into this category. These are very suitable for
teenage or mildly dry skin if it feels tight or slightly uncomfortable
after washing. These preparations are also often marketed as day-
time moisturizing agents for use under make-up.

Moisturizers are valuable for all skin types. The keratinocytes of
the epidermis have a high water content, but a modern environment
in a centrally heated office or home means that moisture is

continually being drawn out of the skin. If the keratinocytes lose some of their water content, small lines appear on the skin and it loses its youthful bloom. Most skins look better and feel more comfortable if a moisturizer is applied in the morning after washing the face. In some dry environments this may need to be re-applied at lunchtime.

Heavier moisturizing and nourishing preparations, containing both moisturizing agents and heavier lipids (oil and grease components) aimed at replacing the body's lost surface sebum, are often marketed as night-time moisturizers or night creams. Another constituent may be a **humectant**—a preparation that attracts moisture to the skin from the surrounding atmosphere.

These heavier moisturizers tend to be thicker creams that are sold in pots rather than in bottles, and leave the skin surface looking slightly shiny and oily. These may make older, drier skin more comfortable but should not be used by teenagers or by anyone with a tendency to acne as they may clog the pilosebaceous follicle openings ('pores') and make the situation worse. A condition known as cosmetically-induced acne is the result of applying excessive grease to the skin. This grease may be found in heavier moisturizing creams and in pomades and greases used to tame curly hair. For this reason cosmetically induced acne can often be seen around the hairline.

SPECIAL INGREDIENTS

Liposomes

Some of the more expensive, heavier night creams and moisturizing creams have very specialized actions and special ingredients. One particular type of ingredient advertized in some of these products are **liposomes**. Liposomes are small spheres that carry lubrication in the form of lipid and fatty, oily material plus water between individual cells on the skin surface down into the deeper cells of the epidermis. Thus, the claims that these liposome-containing preparations can penetrate deeper into the skin than other products may be correct. Remember, however, that all this action is going on within the epidermis and above the basement membrane, so the main value is that they help plump up the keratinocytes in the deeper as well as the more superficial layers of the epidermis, but have no effect on the underlying dermis.

Retin-A

An interesting recent development in the dermatological world has been the publication of reports that a cream containing a form of vitamin A (Retin-A) applied to the skin could literally roll back the years and remove wrinkles from older skin. A number of studies have subsequently been carefully carried out using creams containing small concentrations of this vitamin A-like preparation in highly respected dermatology departments. It appears that regular use of these vitamin A preparations results in the disappearance of both small surface wrinkles and, in some cases, some of the deeper, apparently more permanent skin creases that develop on skin as it gets older.

Some of the volunteers who used these vitamin A preparations on their skin consented to have small skin biopsies taken from their face or arm before and after using the vitamin A preparations for several months. Comparison of the before and after biopsies showed that after a few months of Retin-A treatment the epidermis became thicker, with a larger number of cell layers than was present before. Some studies also made the unexpected discovery that the underlying dermis was thicker and more plumped-up, a picture usually seen in younger skin. This last observation illustrates the difficult borderline area between cosmetics and topical drugs acting on the skin—cosmetics are not meant to penetrate below the epidermis.

However, at the present time it appears that the claims made for vitamin A preparations applied to the skin externally as partial restorers of lost youth are indeed true. It must be stressed that these are creams containing small concentrations of a derivative of vitamin A, and that increasing vitamin A in the diet, taking vitamin A capsules by mouth, or applying vitamin A capsules to the skin, would not have the same effect.

A further important point to bear in mind is that most people who apply Retin-A to their skin find that they can no longer tolerate natural sunlight. For this reason part of the routine of becoming a Retin-A user involves giving up sunbathing completely and using a high SPF sun-screen at all times when out-of-doors in sunny weather. Some dermatologists have suggested that it is this avoidance of sun exposure that is partly responsible for the rejuvenating effect of Retin-A, but examination of the skin with the microscope shows that this is not the whole explanation.

At the time of writing, a number of studies are in progress in many dermatology departments in both Europe and North America to establish the role of Retin-A in various concentrations in disease states, not only for the cosmetic problem of wrinkles. In future it may also have a role to play in the management of actinic keratoses, in stimulating healing in chronic leg ulcers, and in many other conditions. Many dermatologists are very excited about these studies, as not only are they likely to improve the range of treatments available for a wide range of conditions but, at the same time, they are likely to help explain the underlying cause of a number of skin problems—and this in turn could lead to prevention.

MISCELLANEOUS INGREDIENTS IN NOURISHING CREAMS

Many moisturizing and nourishing creams available on the cosmetic counter contain interesting specific ingredients.

VEGETABLE ADDITIVES

An example of a natural vegetable additive is aloe vera. This is a rather interesting cactus-type plant, and there is no doubt that some people find a lotion or cream containing aloe vera extract very soothing after sunburns or scalds from hot water.

There are also preparations containing jojoba oil and avocado oil. The exact method by which any of these special extracts works on the epidermis, if indeed they have a special effect, is not well-established. If, however, a cream or lotion containing such an extract is found to suit the skin, it is highly unlikely to be doing any harm.

COLLAGEN

Collagen is an important component of the deeper part of the skin—the dermis; elastic tissue is also found in this area. The individual molecules of collagen and elastin are large and cannot pass through the epidermis to the underlying dermis. Remember also that if a cream or ointment causes a structural change to the permanent parts of the skin—the basal layer of the epidermis and the dermis—it should be classified as a drug or medicine rather than as a cosmetic. It is likely, therefore, that creams advertized as containing collagen or elastin are mainly doing good because of the effect of their moisture and oil or lipid content on the epidermis, and also because of stimulation of the circulation brought about when these creams are massaged into the skin.

OTHER ADDITIVES

The exact effect on the skin of other, more exotic, materials (for example, royal jelly) found in creams and moisturizers has not been scientifically established. As with many other of the more unusual preparations to be found on the cosmetics counter of the department stores, it is likely that the main benefit will be due to the moisturizing ability of the preparation in question, and to the massaging effect of applying the preparation. This will usually stimulate the flow of blood through the small blood vessels in the skin, and thus bring a clearer, fresher look to the skin surface.

PREPARATIONS FOR SPECIAL SITES

Some of the creams available have been tailor-made for different parts of the skin. For example, there is a wide range of preparations available for the skin around the eye, and special preparations are marketed for the neck. The important point about the skin around the eye is that is unusually thin, and is not firmly tethered to underlying structures. This means that if the skin around the eye is pulled or tugged, for example when applying or removing eye make-up, it is very easy to stretch it and cause small wrinkles. It is therefore particularly important when washing, drying, or touching the face to treat the skin around the eyes delicately.

It is unlikely that any specific preparation applied to the eye area will remove dark circles under the eye or puffiness, as these are caused on the one hand by a poor circulation and lack of sleep, and on the other hand by a slight excess of fluid in that part of the skin. The best way to avoid dark circles under the eyes is to have adequate sleep and to take regular exercise.

Another area of the body for which special creams are marketed is the neck. Many women are aware that the neck skin appears to age more rapidly than the skin on the face, and may wonder if such special preparations are worthwhile. In general the neck is exposed to wind and sunshine as much as the face, but usually with none of the protection applied to the facial skin with make-up or moisturizer. There is no published evidence that neck creams containing ingredients such as collagen or elastin are any better for the neck than a conventional moisturizer. The point to remember is to use a moisturizer on the neck regularly, and to protect the skin of the neck, particularly at the sides, with a sunscreen.

EXFOLIANT AND SCRUB PREPARATIONS

Cleansing scrubs or exfoliant creams generally have a slightly gritty texture, and some contain oatmeal. They are meant to be used after removing surface grime and make-up from the skin, and their function is to remove the most superficial layers of epidermis from the skin, leaving—hopefully—a smoother, perhaps pinker, surface underneath. Remember that dead and worn-out epidermal cells are being shed from the skin surface all the time, and that the simple act of washing the face and patting it dry with a towel has a mild exfoliating action. Exfoliating preparations will speed up this process of shedding our outermost epidermal cells, but in doing so they may also encourage some dryness of the skin. Exfoliating scrubs will do no harm if not used too frequently, but a larger than usual quantity of moisturizing agent should be applied to the skin after their use.

FACE MASKS AND PACKS

A wide range of face masks and face packs are available. Most of these are aimed at 'deep cleansing' the skin and removing surface fat or lipid. Some also have a mild peeling effect and remove the surface layer of epidermis in the same way as the exfoliating scrub preparations. Face packs are mainly aimed at younger, possibly blemished skin and may have a temporary effect, probably mostly in stimulating the skin circulation. Once again, they do no harm

provided they are not used too frequently, when they might dry
the skin up and cause flaking.

In summary, modern skin care preparations can be soothing,
smoothing, and pleasant to use. Used sensibly, they will keep the
skin feeling clean and fresh; a moisturizer is strongly recommended
for daily use whatever your age and sex. However, the skin is part
of the body, and general health and fitness measures will do just as
much to retain healthy, comfortable and pleasant-looking skin as
any specific skin preparation.

The important general health rules as far as the skin (and the rest
of the body) is concerned are:

1. Eat a sensible, balanced diet, including plenty of fresh fruit,
vegetables, and fibre. Healthy skin requires normal intake of all the
natural vitamins. Healthy people on Western diets usually have an
adequate vitamin intake, but if you are concerned that your diet
may be inadequate, a multivitamin pill taken every day may do
some good. If your skin requires vitamins, it generally requires
them taken by mouth and not applied to the skin.

2. Do not aim to lose a lot of weight in a hurry, particularly if
you are aged 40 or over. Sudden loss of weight can make the skin
look drawn and haggard, and can make you look considerably
older than your years. If weight loss is required, it is kinder to the
skin to carry this out gradually, losing only a pound or two per
week over several months, rather than embarking on one of the
more drastic regimes.

3. Have a regular exercise programme, and try to do some of
this out-of-doors; One of the best exercises in the world is
straightforward brisk walking. Try to fit walking, swimming,
cycling or some other regular mild exercise into your daily programme. Skin, like the rest of the body organs benefits from good
circulation of the blood, both to bring necessary nutrients to the
skin surface and to carry the venous blood back to the heart. A
healthy circulation will make the skin look pinker and fresher.

4. Do not smoke. Quite apart from all the other serious effects
smoking has on your health, studies of regular smokers have shown

that the skin of their faces looks older and more lined than the skin of non-smokers of the same age.

5. Be sure you have enough sleep. Chronic tiredness is very ageing.

6. Use a moisturizing preparation daily. Choose a preparation suitable for your age range and your skin type, and remember that you will need to change this preparation as you get older.

7. Be sensible about sun exposure. Enjoy being out-of-doors in fine weather but do not allow the skin to burn, and remember that habitually sun-exposed skin rapidly becomes older-looking. Get into the habit of using a sun-screen in hot sunny weather when you are out-of-doors. Apply this before going out into the sun, and reapply every 2 hours, or after swimming. Buy a comfortable, attractive, broad-brimmed sun hat and *wear* it.

These simple rules will probably do more to maintain the skin in a healthy, comfortable, relatively young-looking condition for a long time than any of the complex skin care regimes and expensive preparations.

10.

Hair and nails

SCALP HAIR

The hair is continually being shed and replaced. We are born with a fixed number of hair follicles on the scalp, and these go through the cycle of growth, shedding, and resting before the cycle recommences and a new young hair grows out.

The hair follicles respond to male and female hormones circulating in the bloodstream. In general, female hormones encourage hair growth, so that during pregnancy a higher proportion than usual of the hair follicles are in the growth phase. Male hormones have a more varied effect but on certain areas of the scalp, particularly the temples and the top of the head, they tend to inhibit hair growth, so that some males lose hair from these sites quite early in life. The tendency of male hair loss tends to run in families and is a result of the hair follicle ceasing to make a long strong terminal hair of the type normally seen on the scalp. Instead, it produces a vellus hair— a small fine downy hair—of the type usually seen on the forearms. At present we do not understand the stimuli that cause this change, and cannot prevent or reverse it but, at the time of writing, a number of scientific research groups are trying to understand the signals that switch the hair follicles on and off. If they succeed, this knowledge may open the door to either prevention or treatment of baldness in males.

Scalp hair varies in its thickness. In general, fair hair is finer and darker hair is thicker, giving a fuller look to the head of hair. No treatment can alter the average thickness of each individual hair, although there are applications that can be used after shampooing to give a temporary impression of a thicker scalp of hair.

As we get older, hair tends to get thinner and more brittle. For this reason, it is important to treat older hair gently, and not to damage it with repeated perms, bleaching, heat or vigorous back combing.

Hair varies greatly in its straightness or tendency to form curls and waves. This feature varies throughout life, and many small children have delightful baby curls that vanish as the child grows. As with skin colour, human beings seem to have a contrary approach to their inborn tendency to straight or curly hair, as can be seen in chemist's shop, where rows of packets of home permanent waving kits can be found next to the hair straighteners!

SHAMPOOS

Shampoo has to remove material that has reached the hair from the environment—grime from the atmosphere—and material from the scalp itself. This is sebum, from the sebaceous glands draining into the hair follicles, sweat, and also the shed layers of the outer part of the epidermis, which are present on the scalp just as in other parts of the body.

Most shampoos are based on detergent that dissolves and removes all these substances. However, if the shampoo contains too high a proportion of detergent, all the lubrication will be stripped off the individual hairs, leaving a clean but dry, brittle, and dull-looking head of hair. For this reason, shampoos contain various percentages of detergent according to whether they are aimed at greasy or dry scalps. In general, teenagers have greasy scalps just as they tend to have a greasier facial skin than older people, and should choose their shampoo accordingly. If, however, as many teenagers do nowadays, they wash their hair every day, then a milder shampoo labelled 'for daily or frequent use' is more appropriate, as these will not dry the hair out too much.

The range of available shampoos is very wide indeed, and the variety of 'special' additional ingredients is vast. As with make-up, trial and error is the best approach to finding the most suitable shampoo.

Healthy hair will remain healthy and shining if it is washed gently with an appropriate shampoo, if no harsh chemicals such as bleach are applied to it, and if it is not exposed to high temperatures either from electrical appliances or strong natural sunlight. The shine of a healthy head of hair is due to the outer part of the hair—the cuticle—reflecting light, and to do this, the strands of hair must be smooth, with no breaks or irregularities, such as split ends. Naturally oily hair, although it may quickly become dull due to dust and dirt collecting on it, generally looks healthy and shiny just after a shampoo with no additional conditioner. This is because the hair's natural oil acts as an in-built conditioner. In contrast, newly washed dry hair often looks rather dull, because all the surface oil has been stripped away. This is one of the reasons for choosing a shampoo that will remove grime, but not all the natural lubricating and shine-producing oil. Straight hair usually looks shinier than curly hair, because the smoothness of a straight hair shaft reflects more light.

Modern life-styles are not usually kind to hair. Many people have their hair permed, bleached or both. An even larger number wash their hair frequently, perhaps daily, and then dry it with a blow drier, or use tongs or other electrical appliances such as heated rollers. As a result of all this, hair is being subjected to stresses and strains that cause the normally smooth outer surface of the individual hairs, the cuticle, to become roughened and damaged. Individual hairs may also break off, giving rise to split ends. These problems can be reduced, by limiting the amount of damage done to hair. For example, both perms and bleaching damage hair, so choose one or other, but not both. Choose a hairstyle that does not depend on the regular daily use of a hot hair drier or tongs, and keep these appliances for occasional rather than daily use. If a hairdrier is necessary to save time in the morning, read the manufacturer's instructions, and keep the nozzle at the recommended distance from the scalp and, although drying the hair will take a little longer, choose a warm rather than hot setting for everyday use.

CONDITIONERS

In addition to these suggestions, you may wish to use a conditioner to improve the look and feel of your hair. Basically, conditioners act by smoothing down the outer cuticle of the hair shaft. Conditioners that contain small molecules of protein may even temporarily repair damage to individual hairs. Conditioners also reduce static electricity in hair, and prevent it from flying about.

Conditioners come in two main groups—the quick-to-use rinse off immediately type and the heavier variety to be left in contact with the hair for 20 minutes, often also with a hot towel applied over the top. There are also shampoos available whch claim to both cleanse and condition at the same time, but as the two actions are not entirely compatible it is usually more effective to use a shampoo and conditioner separately.

Teenagers and young adults who have unpermed, uncoloured, and non-bleached hair are unlikely to require to use conditioners regularly. This may not be true for those who have long hair, as the individual hairs may have become 'weathered' and slightly damaged in the course of growth. A conditioner will improve the appearance of hairs damaged in this way. In general conditioners make hair soft and floppier—more difficult to set in a firm style. With strong, wiry hair this may be a positive advantage, but baby-fine hair will become even more difficult to style. The way in which hair conditioners work can perhaps be compared to fabric conditioners, in that both are designed to coat and smooth rough fibres.

It is possible to use too much conditioner. This will not damage the hair in any way, but it will become lank and limp. This happens most rapidly with fine hair, which can become very flat and lose all body when too much conditioner, particularly heavy conditioner is applied to the hair. There are shampoos that can be used to strip off this build-up of conditioner.

Conditioning rinses, cream rinses, and blow-drying lotions

These preparations can all be thought of as dilute or mild conditioners. They contain the same ingredients—mainly materials called **quaternary ammonium compounds**—aimed at smoothing the hair shaft and reducing static. Rinses are washed out of the hair before drying but blow-dry lotion is left on the hair. Their function is to protect the shaft of the hair from the heat and traction involved in blow-drying. They do appear to help in preventing damage to the hair, but are not as effective as the heavier conditioners in this respect.

Trial and error will be needed before deciding upon suitable conditioning products. A few general words of advice may, however, be helpful. Teenagers do not usually need heavy conditioners, which will make their scalps feel even oilier than is already the case, and may make their hair look very lank. However, a perm or a bleaching treatment at any age should be followed by a conditioner for several shampoos after having this done, as most of these processes do cause some damage to the hair.

Conditioners are also often needed during and after a sunny summer holiday because both strong sunshine and salt water cause drying of the hair and splitting of the ends of the individual hairs. However, over-application, for example a conditioner followed by a cream rinse followed by a blow drying lotion, will result in a flat, lank, dull head of hair.

PERMS, BLEACHES, AND COLOURINGS

The basic principle behind perming lotions is to alter the bonds or links in the hair between the units of protein, the amino acids, of which the hairs are constructed. Thus when a perm is 'taking', the actual structure of the hair is altered, and the result is that the hair is more brittle and porous until the permed hair grows out. Therefore, permed hair requires more care, with regular use of a conditioner and protection from heat.

Further sources of damage to chemically altered hair are sea water and chlorinated water in swimming pools. Everyone, but particularly those with permed, bleached, or coloured hair should rinse their hair with fresh water after swimming in the sea or in a chlorinated pool.

Bleaches and 'highlighters' also involve causing physical changes to the structure of the hair and once again, hair that has been treated in this way requires special care. Bleached hair often becomes very dry and straw-like, or even changes colour if exposed to strong sunlight—a sun-hat or scarf will prevent this.

The combination of perming and bleaching or colouring is a particularly tricky one and should be done by a professional hairdresser, who will advise on which procedure to carry out first and will work hard at reconditioning the hair afterwards; this combination is not one to embark upon as a do-it-yourself project at home.

If a temporary or semi-permanent colouring rinse is to be used on unpermed hair at home, the manufacturer's instructions should be read carefully and followed to the letter. The great majority will recommend a test or trial area on a small strand of hair to make sure that you are not allergic to any of the ingredients. This is good advice and will prevent those with such an allergy developing a red, painful, swollen face and scalp.

SETTING AGENTS—SPRAYS, GELS, AND MOUSSES

These agents are designed to give fine hair body, and to help the hair retain the shape in which it was styled or set for longer. They coat the hair shafts with a fine resin, which acts like a mild glue in temporarily holding the hairs, and thus the style, together. They generally make newly washed hair look tidier, but tend to attract dust and grease, so that the hair tends to look dull and flat within a day or two. As with conditioners, it is possible to over-use these agents and make individual hairs look and feel coated, dull, and sticky. These preparations should be used sparingly, and the hair will need fairly frequent shampooing because they all tend to make it feel and look rather tired and flat.

The great majority of hair care preparations contain fragrances. Individuals with a perfume allergy will need to select their hair products carefully. The Simple range of products is useful because they are fragrance-free, but many of the 'natural ingredient' ranges contain added fragrances, and need therefore to be avoided by those who have an allergy to fragrances.

DANDRUFF

Dandruff is simply an excessive and visible shedding of the super-ficial cornified layers of the epidermis of the scalp. For some individuals it is a continuing minor problem and makes dark blouses or jackets, on which the dandruff scales stand out, a social hazard. There is at present some evidence to suggest that dandruff is associated with the presence in the hair follicles of large numbers of a yeast organism called *Pityrosporon*. This yeast is found on most scalps, but in some dandruff sufferers the numbers present are much greater than average.

Anti-dandruff shampoos are available and approach the problem in a variety of ways. The most common is the addition of a mild antiseptic agent or an antifungal, which reduces the numbers of *Pityrosporon*. These antiseptic-containing shampoos can be bought over the counter in a chemist's shop but most of the antifungal shampoos require a doctor's prescription in the UK. (eg Nizoral shampoo).

A second approach is to apply a cream containing a **keratolytic**—a preparation that lifts this scale away from the scalp—overnight before shampooing. The scale will build up again but, for a day or two, the shoulders will be clear of dandruff scales.

TEMPORARY THINNING OF THE SCALP HAIR

A number of situations are associated with a temporary thinning of
the hair, which is usually caused by a larger than usual proportion
of the hairs being in the resting or shedding stage, and not in the
growing stage. In younger women this is commonly seen 3–6
months after the birth of a baby, and the problem may persist for
another 3–4 months.

At any age there is often a temporary shedding of hair after
severe illness, particularly if this has been associated with high
fevers. The technical term for this is **telogen effluvium**. Time will
remedy the situation and the normal pattern of hair growth will
resume.

Those who are on chemotherapy for serious illnesses may
experience loss of scalp hair because some, but not all, drugs used
in chemotherapy affect the growing hair follicle. Once again,
normal hair growth will return when the chemotherapy is stopped.

In addition to these situations, certain illnesses associated with
parts of the body other than the skin may be associated with poor
scalp hair growth. These include disorders of the thyroid gland and,
in some people, severe anaemia due to loss of iron. In both of these
examples the hair will recover when the underlying problem is
treated.

MORE PERMANENT THINNING OF THE SCALP HAIR

In our society it is acceptable for men to lose scalp hair and,
although some such men may disagree, film stars and olympic
swimmers have demonstrated that total loss of male scalp hair can
be attractive, and certainly not hamper a successful career in the
public eye. For women, however, the situation is different and even
thinning of the hair is felt to be socially unacceptable. Most women
do not noticeably lose their scalp hair, but a few develop thinning
on the top of the scalp. This usually happens after the menopause,
and can be very distressing. At present there are studies in progress
to decide whether or not a lotion—minoxidil—applied daily to the
scalp can help delay or prevent this problem. In men, minoxidil
appears to delay the development of male pattern baldness, but
only for as long as the lotion is being rubbed daily on to the scalp.
In other words, this is a treatment for life. In the UK this type of

hair loss is not regarded as an illness, and therefore minoxidil cannot be obtained on a National Health Service prescription, but only on private prescription. People who are concerned by this type of hair loss should discuss with their doctor or dermatologist whether or not they feel sufficiently strongly about the hair loss to commit themselves indefinitely to a daily treatment regime, and also to the cost involved.

KEEPING THE HAIR AS HEALTHY AS POSSIBLE

Hairstyles should be realistic for the hair type, whether this is soft and fine or springy and curly. Perms, bleaches, and artificial colourings should be used with the advice of an expert hairdresser and only one such treatment should be used at a time. Remember that however 'kind' to the hair they are said to be on the advertisement, they all damage the actual structure of the hair to a greater or lesser extent.

An appropriate shampoo should be used as often as the hair appears to need it, and should always be thoroughly rinsed out. Hair-dryers and other heated appliances should not be used more than once or twice a week—direct heat applied to the hair causes damage. If possible, opt for a hairstyle that can be left to dry naturally.

An appropriate conditioner should be used if the hair is dry and dull-looking, if there are split ends or after a lot of sun and sea water.

HEAD LICE AND NITS

Many people associate head lice with a lack of cleanliness or personal hygiene; this is emphatically not the case. Head lice can move in on an impeccably clean scalp and, unless the subject is discussed sensibly and openly, and prevention and treatment measures are well publicized, the problem will continue to smoulder on.

Head lice are a species of louse with a preference for the human scalp. Their eggs are called nits. One head louse can lay very large numbers of eggs, and tends to do this on the hair shafts closest to the scalp, as the louse appears to be more comfortable at the higher temperatures found closer to the scalp. This is why, when examining a scalp for signs of infestation, it is important to check the area near the scalp very thoroughly. It is unusual to see a head louse on the scalp, but the eggs or nits can be identified in large numbers if one knows what to look for. They seem to have a preference for long, fine, straight hair and are most commonly found in the hair behind the ears or at the nape of the neck. They usually cause no initial discomfort, so the sufferer will be unaware of the problem but, as time goes by, and if the scalp is not treated, the area will become itchy and infected. If the scalp is examined the impression is that there are some flakes of dandruff sticking to the hairs, usually an inch or two from the actual scalp. On closer inspection it will be seen that these little white flecks—the nits—are firmly stuck on to the hair shaft. If not removed, each nit will, after an incubation period, hatch out into a new young louse, and the whole cycle will begin again.

Head lice are generally transmitted from scalp to scalp by fairly prolonged, close, head contact. Thus, the playground and the family are the likely places for transmission to take place. The lice require body warmth to survive and therefore do not last long on combs or hats, despite popular myths that this is how they travel. From time to time, there are outbreaks of head louse infection, often running through a large number of children in a primary school class. Health visitors and others may visit the school and eradicate the majority of cases, but reinfection may occur. It is generally believed that children are at greater risk than adults of acquiring head lice, but a possible source of reinfection is a senior member of the family, perhaps a grandmother.

If head lice or nits are suspected in a child, ask the school nurse, local pharmacist, doctor or dermatologist to confirm the suspicion, as it can sometimes be surprisingly difficult to distinguish between specks of dandruff and nits. The treatment recommended by the pharmacist, school nurse or health visitor should be carried out and the scalps of all family members or close family friends who come into contact with the child should be checked. This may at first seem an embarrassing problem to discuss openly with friends and relations, but unless it is accepted as a fairly common and minor problem, which can affect even the cleanest of scalps, the cycle of reinfection will continue. Once all sufferers have been identified and treatment has been arranged, the child's school should be contacted, so that any classroom problems can also be identified and treated.

Treatment involves using an insecticide or acaricide preparation containing malathion, carbaryl or phenothrin, leaving it in contact with the hair for 12 hours, and then painstakingly combing out the dead and now harmless nits with a fine comb. The local chemist can often supply both the material and advice on how to deal with this problem. Acaricides can be absorbed through the skin and cause side-effects, but only if used in excessive amounts or left on the scalp for too long, or used on the scalps of infants. If the instructions are followed carefully they will do no harm.

BODY HAIR

There are striking cultural differences in the attitude to removal of hair from the legs, armpits, and other areas. If removal is considered desirable, shaving, waxing, and the use of depilatory creams containing thioglycolates are all effective. These act by causing the hair shafts to swell up and become irretrievably damaged.

Some, usually dark-haired, women are concerned about what they feel to be excessive hair growth on other body sites, such as the face, the forearms, and the breasts. There are large variations in what is regarded as normal as far as body hair is concerned, and those of southern European ancestry may have more visible body hair than a fair-haired Scandinavian or a Scot. Usually, there is no real difference in the actual amount of hair, but the fact that it is dark rather than fair makes it much more obvious. In Mediterranean countries and in hispanic communities in North America the visibility of this body hair is entirely normal, but in northern Europe or the northern US individuals may become very concerned and embarrassed about their body hair because they feel it is socially unacceptable.

Although excess body hair is occasionally associated with hormonal problems, this is unusual, and the great majority of women who are referred to dermatologists for investigation of a medical cause of possible excess hair have no hormonal abnormality. They may still, however, want to reduce what they perceive as too much body hair.

For problems on the face, waxing and bleaching are both useful and if the problem is that of only a few coarser than average hairs around the chin, plucking with tweezers can be quite effective. The advantage of waxing is that the hairs are removed from below the level of the skin surface, so although it is mildly uncomfortable at the time, waxing need not be repeated as often as other methods of hair removal. Some women who wax areas of their face feel that the newly waxed areas have a 'bald' appearance compared with the normal growth of fine downy hair elsewhere, but the differences are usually very silght and only visible to someone looking very closely.

Many dark-haired women find that the alternative of bleaching the hair on their face is a useful camouflage method, as fair hair is never as obvious as dark hair.

Depilatory creams, even those labelled as specifically for facial use, often cause some irritation, and should be used with caution if at all.

ELECTROLYSIS

Electrolysis is not generally available in the National Health Service, but many women who feel that they have a problem with superfluous hair may consider this method of hair removal.

The basic principle is that an electric current passed down the hair follicle destroys the actual growing part of the hair root from which new hairs develop. Thus, no new hair will develop after successful treatment to that follicle. Every individual hair follicle must be treated, and this is extremely time-consuming. On average, it may be possible to treat 2 square inches in a 30 minute session. Thus, electrolysis is not only time-consuming, but also expensive. If not carried out by an experienced and qualified operator, there is the possibility of minor scarring. For electrolysis to be successful reasonably long hairs must be present and, after treatment, the area will be red for a day or two while the skin settles down.

It is wise to find an operator who is a member of the Institute of Electrolysis, and to ask for a preliminary consultation to discuss the area to be treated, the time it will take, and the cost before deciding to undergo electrolysis. Many good electrolysists will also recommend speaking to someone who is nearing the end of a course of treatment, to obtain their opinion of the treatment.

Prescribable medical treatments are available for excessive hair growth. These are occasionally used, once the doctor has carried out appropriate tests to confirm that there is no underlying hormonal illness.

One of these is an anti-androgen preparation called **cyproterone**, which is always prescribed with an essential oral contraceptive because a pregnancy commenced while on cyproterone could result in feminization of a male baby. The trade-name for one such combination is Dianette.

These preparations must be taken for 6–9 months before significant improvement can be expected, and continuous use for longer than 12–18 months is not advised because of side-effects, which include breast tenderness and cyst formation. There are therefore only a short-term measure for a limited number of women.

There is no doubt that the idea of excess body hair is a very emotive and psychologically disturbing problem for many women, but often the problem, or perceived problem, which appears very serious to the person involved, may be barely visible to everyone else. It is a good idea to discuss such problems with a good friend or relative, who will give an honest opinion, rather than bottling the problem up to affect everyday life. It is highly likely that the problem has got out of perspective.

THE NAILS

In general, nails cause fewer problems than hair, but when problems do arise in the nail or around it, there may be a lot of pain. This is particularly true if infection or bleeding develops under the nail, as the material in this site may become trapped, and exert a lot of pressure on sensitive nerves.

Like hair, nail can be thought of as modified epidermis. The underlying nail bed is the dermis and has a very rich blood supply. The growing end of the nail is the area under the nail fold. The finger-nails take about 6 months to grow out from this area to the free edge and the toe-nails take even longer—about 2 years. Nails grow more rapidly in the summer than in the winter, and faster in younger people.

The cuticle is a thin membrane dividing the nail from the skin of the nail fold. It is not a useless piece of modified skin to be prised off by harsh manicuring tools, but has an important function in preventing infection, dirt, or debris lodging in the narrow space between nail and nailfold.

Normal healthy nails need no special care other than regular trimming. Both finger- and toe-nails should be cut straight across and, particularly on the toes, should not be curved around the end of the digit. A curved, free nail end will encourage the development of an ingrowing nail, which digs into the adjacent finger, or more often toe, and can be extremely painful. Like skin, nails react badly to immersion in strong degreasing detergents and vinyl gloves and regular use of a hand cream are good practice.

Common minor problems with nails are splitting, ridging, and white marks. Splitting due to thin nails may be due to an inherited tendency, but may also occur if the diet is low in protein. The best way to cure this is to eat more protein. The nail cannot absorb protein through its surface, so applying protein-rich lotions will not be useful. In the past it has been suggested that gelatine would strengthen nails if eaten regularly. I am not aware of any true scientific evidence showing that gelatine is better than any other type of protein in helping nails grow, but as it is an easy and convenient source of protein, it could be tried. Alternatively, intake of the major protein-containing foods—meat, fish, eggs, and cheese—could be increased. Whichever method is tried, because of the length of time nails take to grow, it will be at least 3 months before any obvious benefit is seen. Ridged nails and white marks on nails may be due to trauma to the nails, for example over-enthusiastic manicuring—treat the nails gently, particularly around the cuticle area.

Common minor problems with nails include warts around the nails (**periungual warts**), **paronychia**, and fungal infection of the nails, which generally has spread from the adjacent skin.

A rarer but potentially very important problem is the development of malignant melanoma in the nail bed—a brown or black pigmented mark under or around the nail should be checked by a doctor.

PERIUNGUAL WARTS

These are common warts (as discussed already on p. 34) that involve the skin around the nail. Because the skin in this area is relatively bound down to surrounding structures, the warts can press on nerves and can therefore be painful. If not treated they may cause the nail to grow in an abnormal manner. They should therefore be treated sooner rather than later.

PARONYCHIA

Paronychia is inflammation around the nail and is usually the result of infection in the narrow space between the nail and the nail fold; it is associated with loss of cuticle. Individuals at greatest risk are those who have their hands in water a lot but find it difficult to use waterproof gloves, for example nurses and individuals who handle food, such as bakers. Paronychia can be recognized by the presence around the nail of a tender, often throbbing, raised red margin. Sometimes a little bead of pus can be seen or pressed out of the nail fold area. The infection may be bacterial or fungal, particularly with an organism called *Candida*, which grows well in the moist environment around the nail. The infection is often due to a mixture of these micro-organisms.

Paronychia requires careful attention. The doctor or dermatologist can prescribe appropriate preparations, but the way in which these are used is important. It is also necessary to try to keep the hands out of water, or the problem is likely to return. Ointments and lotions for this problem require to be coaxed and massaged carefully into the crevice between the nail and nail fold to ensure that the medication reaches its target. Once the paronychia has been cured, the cuticle should be allowed to grow back to perform its protective role. If paronychia has gone untreated for any length of time the nail itself may be ridged and damaged. This will come right in time, but this will take months not weeks.

TINEA UNGUIUM

This name describes infection of the nails by the same organisms—the dermatophytes—that cause athlete's foot. The problem usually develops months after the itchy, peeling skin between the toes. The usual signs that the nails are infected are that they become crumbly, ridged, and in time may become very heaped up and misshapen. This can reach the stage of causing problems with footwear. Any number of nails may become involved in this way.

Prevention is the best way to deal with **tinea unguium**. Athlete's foot (see p. 51) should be treated promptly. It is easy to cure when confined to the skin, but much more difficult to remove the problem from the toe-nails. If the infection spreads to the nails, creams and ointments are at present ineffective, and a course of antifungal tablets will be required. These are usually effective in clearing infection from one or two finger-nails but need to be taken for 3–6 months. This optimism is not justified in the case of toe-nails and, even if the tablets are taken for a year or more (and this will be necessary because toe-nails grow so slowly), the infection frequently persists. At present, trials are being carried out on a new antifungal drug that may change this rather gloomy picture over the next year or two.

As with skin, the best treatment for healthy nails is to keep them clean and dry, and to apply a little lubrication in the form of a rich hand cream or special nail cream, although the ingredients of the latter are almost identical to those found in hand creams. The most vulnerable part of the nail is between the hard nail itself and the skin. This is the area partly protected by the cuticle, so do not damage or destroy this protective membrane.

NAIL COSMETICS

Most modern nail varnishes do no harm, but some of the varnish removers are very drying and hard on the nails. If over-used they can lead to dryness, brittleness, and splitting of the nails. Always wash the nails thoroughly after applying nail varnish remover, and then rub in a rich hand cream.

While artificial nails may be regarded by some as either fun or glamorous for special occasions, the glue used to stick them on is not particularly kind to the underlying real nail. Artificial nails can therefore cause damage and should not be used all the time.

11.

Summary and thoughts for the future

A healthy-looking skin is an important part of the body image. This is evident when an already-self-conscious teenager develops a spot, but skin problems at any age can affect confidence and our sense of well-being. Modern treatment for skin diseases has come a very long way in the past decade, but clearly prevention is better than cure, and a high proportion of skin problems can be prevented, as I hope I have emphasized in this book.

Over the next 10 years I would predict an even greater understanding about keeping the skin healthy-looking throughout life and preventing the ageing changes brought about by exposure to the sun. Again, however, prevention must be better than cure and adoption of at least some of the approaches suggested in Chapter 7 is necessary. I would also predict that more effective treatments will become available for common problems such as psoriasis and eczema, although the availability of a totally effective treatment free from side-effects may not be possible. Again, however, I predict that prevention may have a part to play in these disorders once we understand the exact cause of the disease in question.

Appendix

List of useful organizations

National Eczema Society
4 Tavistock Place
London WC1H 9RA
UK

Psoriasis Association (branches worldwide)
7 Milton Street
Northampton NN2 7JG
UK

Index

144   Index